Overcome Anxiety Book

CRAFTED BY SKRIUWER

Copyright © 2024 by Skriuwer.

All rights reserved. No part of this book may be used or reproduced in any form whatsoever without written permission except in the case of brief quotations in critical articles or reviews.

For more information, contact : **kontakt@skriuwer.com** (www.skriuwer.com)

TABLE OF CONTENTS

CHAPTER 1: UNDERSTANDING ANXIETY

- *Seeing anxiety as more than normal stress*
- *Differences between short-term tension and ongoing worry*
- *Myths about anxiety and how it truly works*

CHAPTER 2: SIGNS AND SYMPTOMS

- *Physical clues (racing heart, sweating, muscle tension)*
- *Emotional signs (restlessness, irritability, fear)*
- *Behavioral signals (avoidance, fidgeting, seeking reassurance)*

CHAPTER 3: POSSIBLE CAUSES

- *Brain chemistry and genetic factors*
- *Childhood events and learned patterns*
- *Modern lifestyle and technology influences*

CHAPTER 4: NEGATIVE THINKING PATTERNS

- *Common thinking traps (all-or-nothing, catastrophizing)*
- *Spotting and challenging harmful thoughts*
- *Replacing negative loops with balanced views*

CHAPTER 5: SELF-TALK

- *How inner dialogue shapes mood and confidence*
- *Turning harsh self-talk into kindness*
- *Practical exercises for building positive mental chatter*

CHAPTER 6: STRESS MANAGEMENT

- Identifying daily stressors
- Breathing, relaxation, and time-out methods
- Preventing burnout through balanced routines

CHAPTER 7: DIET AND EXERCISE

- Foods that support a calmer mind
- Managing energy levels and blood sugar
- How regular movement helps ease worry

CHAPTER 8: SLEEP AND RELAXATION

- Importance of restful sleep for mental health
- Nighttime anxiety tips and bedtime routines
- Relaxation drills for day and night

CHAPTER 9: HEALTHY ROUTINES

- Structuring your day to reduce worry
- Morning, afternoon, and evening habits for stability
- Adapting routines to fit personal needs

CHAPTER 10: PANIC AND FEAR

- What panic attacks are and how they start
- Immediate steps to calm the body and mind
- Long-term methods for taming strong fears

CHAPTER 11: SOCIAL ANXIETY

- Why social events can trigger anxiety
- Tools for handling group settings or one-on-one chats
- Building social skills with gradual exposure

CHAPTER 12: ANXIETY AT WORK AND SCHOOL

- Managing deadlines and performance pressure
- Dealing with classroom or meeting anxiety
- Balancing tasks with mental well-being

CHAPTER 13: MINDSET AND BEHAVIOR

- The link between beliefs and actions
- Changing habits that fuel anxiety
- Growing a flexible, positive outlook

CHAPTER 14: LONG-TERM STRATEGIES

- Why short-term fixes are not enough
- Maintaining a healthy life rhythm
- Adapting to future challenges without losing ground

CHAPTER 15: MEDICATION AND THERAPY

- Different types of medication and how they help
- Overview of therapy approaches (CBT, DBT, etc.)
- Combining professional help with self-care tools

CHAPTER 16: BREAKING HARMFUL HABITS

- Recognizing habits that raise anxiety
- Replacements and coping techniques
- Handling withdrawal, temptation, and setbacks

CHAPTER 17: FINDING STRENGTH

- Identifying personal power in daily life
- Overcoming doubt and seeing past successes
- Building resilience through honesty and self-encouragement

CHAPTER 18: DEALING WITH UNCERTAINTY

- *Why the unknown triggers worry*
- *Shifting your view of unpredictable events*
- *Staying calm when outcomes are unclear*

CHAPTER 19: GIVING AND RECEIVING SUPPORT

- *Asking for help without shame*
- *Helping others with empathy and healthy boundaries*
- *Using community or professional resources*

CHAPTER 20: MAINTAINING PROGRESS

- *Spotting early signs of slipping back*
- *Keeping routines fresh and effective*
- *Planning for the future with steady self-care*

CHAPTER 1: UNDERSTANDING ANXIETY

Anxiety is a feeling of worry or nervousness. It can show up when we think something bad might happen. Many people think that anxiety is just simple stress, but it can be much more. It can cause upset thoughts, tense muscles, and other problems in the body. Sometimes anxiety shows up in small ways, like feeling shy at a party. Other times it can become so big that it stops a person from going to work, studying, or spending time with friends. This chapter will look at what anxiety is, why it happens, how it might feel, and some ideas about how to handle it in everyday life.

What Is Anxiety?

Anxiety is more than just feeling uneasy. It can involve many physical and mental signs. The mind might cycle through worries. The body can become tense, and the person might feel restless. This happens for many reasons. Some people are born with a brain that reacts strongly to threats. Others grow up in an environment with high stress levels. When this stress becomes too strong or sticks around for a long time, anxiety can grow.

One main difference between normal stress and anxiety is how it stays in a person's life. Normal stress can be solved by finishing tasks or solving the main problem. Anxiety can linger. It might show up even if nothing scary is happening. This can be confusing. A person might say, "I don't know why I'm so worried." Anxiety can also affect the way people think about themselves. For example, someone might believe they are not good enough because they feel anxious a lot.

Some people think anxiety only affects the mind. But the body can also be affected. Muscles might tighten. Breathing might become shallow. Some people feel dizzy or get headaches. Others might have upset stomachs. The person might not realize these changes are from anxiety, but they often are. Over time, repeated worry can become a pattern that is hard to break.

Anxiety can be seen as the body's alarm system. When it works well, it alerts people to real threats, like touching a hot stove. But when the alarm is too sensitive, it can go off for no real reason. This can lead to discomfort and fear. Learning to calm this alarm is a key step in handling anxiety.

How Anxiety Can Start

Anxiety can have different starting points. One reason can be genetics. Studies show that certain families have more anxious members. If a parent has anxiety, it can raise the chance of children having anxiety, but it's not guaranteed. Another reason is life events. Things like losing a close relative, serious accidents, or repeated stress can trigger high worry. Stressful situations can change how a person sees the world. They might become more watchful. They might scan the environment for bad things that could happen.

Technology also plays a part. With nonstop news and social media, the brain often receives alarming information. Seeing scary headlines can bring a sense of fear. Reading or hearing about upsetting situations can make someone think such events will happen to them too. Over time, this can boost worry.

Personal beliefs can increase anxiety. For example, if someone believes they must be perfect in all tasks, they might feel anxious when they make mistakes. If they see any setback as a disaster, then normal events become sources of stress. These beliefs can push a person to always be on guard, which can make anxiety stronger.

Some people learn to worry from those around them. If they grew up in a household with a lot of tension, they might feel that worry is normal. If they often heard comments like, "Be careful or something bad will happen," they may develop long-term fear. This can happen without the person knowing it.

Worry Patterns

It is useful to recognize the patterns linked to anxiety. One pattern is constant "what if?" thinking. This means a person imagines many bad outcomes. They might think, "What if I fail this test?" or "What if I get sick?" or "What if my friend stops liking me?" A stream of these thoughts can create a chain reaction of worry. The person may not realize they are doing it, but these questions keep the mind unsettled.

Another pattern is overestimating danger. This happens when someone believes that problems are more likely or more severe than they really are. For instance, they might think that a tiny error at work will get them fired. Or a slight pain in the body might seem like a deadly disease. This pattern can worsen anxiety because the person feels that everyday events are big dangers.

Some people with anxiety also avoid things that seem scary. They think avoidance will keep them safe. However, avoiding certain situations can make anxiety stick around. For example, a person might avoid crossing bridges because they fear bridges will collapse. By staying away, they never see that crossing a bridge is safe. As a result, the fear stays and might become stronger.

The Role of the Body

Anxiety not only affects thoughts but also the body. When we feel anxious, hormones like adrenaline are released. These hormones cause the heart to beat faster, muscles to tense, and senses to be on alert. This is sometimes called the "fight or flight" response. In real danger, this response helps us survive by getting us ready to act. But in everyday life, this response can happen even if there is no actual threat.

Some people notice that their stomach hurts when they are anxious. Others might feel their legs shake or their skin sweat. Certain people might breathe faster than usual, leading to lightheadedness. The body might also produce a sense of dread. This physical reaction makes it seem as if something bad is about to happen, even when the situation is safe.

Learning about these body signs is very helpful. By realizing that tense muscles or a racing heart might be connected to anxiety, a person can learn strategies to calm themselves. Techniques like slow breathing or gentle muscle stretching can reduce the body's reaction and send a signal to the mind that things are safe. This helps create a cycle of calm instead of a cycle of fear.

Anxiety and Thinking

The mind and body are closely linked. When a person sees that their body is tense, they might think, "I must be in danger." Then they might scan the environment for threats. If they don't find a threat, they may still feel uneasy. This cycle can keep going until they learn to recognize the pattern and use strategies to manage it.

For many people with anxiety, thoughts can become negative. They might think, "I can't handle this," or "I'm not strong enough." These thoughts can create more anxiety. But thoughts are not always facts. Sometimes they are guesses. When the mind is tense, it might guess in the worst way possible. Learning to spot these guesses can help a person see if they are accurate or if they are just being driven by worry.

Common Myths About Anxiety

1. **Myth: Anxiety is not serious.**
   Truth: Anxiety can make it hard to function. It might affect school, work, or family life.
2. **Myth: Anxiety is a choice.**
   Truth: People do not choose to feel anxious. It can come from complex reasons, including brain chemistry and life events.
3. **Myth: Anxiety will just go away on its own.**
   Truth: While some episodes are short, many cases need attention. Without changes, anxiety may grow worse.
4. **Myth: Only shy people get anxious.**
   Truth: Anxiety can affect anyone, no matter how outgoing they are. It can also show up in different forms.
5. **Myth: Anxiety is the same for everyone.**
   Truth: People have different triggers and feelings. One person might feel panic attacks, while another might worry quietly.

The Influence of Outside Factors

Outside factors can shape anxiety. For instance, a person's work life might involve high demands, long hours, or tough coworkers. This can raise anxiety levels. If someone doesn't have a support system, they might feel they have to handle everything alone. This can make them feel more overwhelmed.

Home life can also add to anxiety. Conflicts, financial problems, or health issues can put a strain on the mind. A calm environment can help ease anxiety, but a tense environment can make it grow. Over time, the person might associate their home with worry and stress. This can cause a cycle of uneasy feelings even when they try to rest.

Social media can add to anxiety. Comparing oneself to others can create feelings of not being good enough. Some people post only their best moments online, which may lead others to think they must also be perfect at all times. This can put extra pressure on people who already feel worried.

Different Types of Anxiety

It's good to note that anxiety comes in many forms:

- **Generalized Anxiety**: Lasting and widespread worry about many things.

- **Social Fear**: Feeling stressed in social situations or worrying about being judged.
- **Phobias**: Strong fear of specific things, like spiders or heights.
- **Panic Attacks**: Sudden feelings of severe fear, often with physical signs such as a racing heart or shortness of breath.
- **Health Anxiety**: Worry about having a serious illness.

Each type might look different, but they often share certain features. A person might feel restlessness, have trouble sleeping, or find it hard to concentrate. They might also notice a jumpy feeling in their body.

Approaches to Understanding Anxiety

To understand anxiety, it can help to look at the thoughts, the emotions, and the body's reaction. One basic way is to keep a simple journal. When someone feels anxious, they can write down the situation, the thoughts going through their mind, and how their body feels. Over time, patterns might appear. The person may see that they feel anxious before big events or when they think about certain topics. They might also see that certain actions or thoughts make them feel worse.

It is also important to understand that anxiety is not just "in the head." It can be influenced by a person's physical health. Things like blood sugar levels, hormone imbalances, or a lack of vitamins can worsen anxiety. That means a complete approach might include a visit to a doctor to rule out any medical causes.

Having good information about anxiety is very helpful. Knowing that anxiety is a body-mind cycle can help a person feel less guilty or ashamed. They might see it as a common but tough condition that can be managed with the right steps. This can make it easier to look for help or follow new strategies.

History and Anxiety

People have likely felt anxiety since ancient times. Early humans had to deal with wild animals and constant danger, so they needed a strong alarm system to keep them alert. Today, some of those alarm signals still remain, even though modern life usually has fewer immediate dangers like wild predators. But the human brain can't always tell if a threat is real or imagined. This can cause a sense of fear that does not match the actual situation.

In many cultures, anxiety has been seen in different ways. Some ancient texts talk about worry of bad luck or punishment. In modern times, we have scientific methods to measure and study anxiety. We now know that anxiety has many aspects, including genetic, mental, and social. This knowledge has led to many ideas for how to manage it.

When Anxiety Becomes Too Much

A certain amount of worry can be useful. For instance, if you have a test tomorrow, a small level of worry might help you study. But if the worry is so strong that you cannot open your books, it becomes a problem. If anxiety stops you from leaving the house, meeting friends, or doing normal tasks, that is a sign it has gotten too big.

Some people with very high anxiety might feel a sense of doom all the time. They might have trouble getting out of bed because everything seems too hard. They might even have racing thoughts at night, making it impossible to sleep. It can help to notice these signs early and take steps to handle them before they grow.

Healthy Ways to See Anxiety

It is important to see anxiety as a problem that can be addressed. It's not a permanent mark on one's character. For example, saying, "I have anxiety" does not mean a person is bad or weak. It means they are dealing with a challenge that can be managed by learning new ways to think and act.

Some people think if they admit to anxiety, others will judge them. But many individuals deal with anxiety. It's one of the most common mental health conditions worldwide. Understanding that anxiety is widespread can help reduce stigma. It can also help people see the benefit of discussing anxiety openly with friends, family, or experts.

Specific Life Stages

Anxiety can show up at different life stages. Children might show anxiety by clinging to parents or crying when they have to go to school. Teenagers might show it by avoiding social events. Adults might show it by overworking or trying to do everything perfectly. Older adults might worry more about health or money. Each stage can have different triggers, but the core sense of fear or dread is the same.

This shows that the roots of anxiety can form early. If a person learns healthy ways to cope when they are young, they might have fewer issues as they grow older. But even if someone did not learn these ways before, it is never too late. The adult brain can still pick up new skills, and people can find relief at any age.

Effects on Relationships

Anxiety can affect how a person interacts with others. They might worry about being judged or disliked. This can cause them to avoid social events or keep their thoughts bottled up. On the other side, they might seek constant reassurance from family or friends. This can strain relationships if the anxious person needs too much comfort or if loved ones do not understand what is happening.

Also, anxiety can lead to anger or frustration. When a person feels on edge, they might snap at others without meaning to. This can lead to guilt or shame later. Over time, this can damage friendships or family bonds. Learning how to communicate feelings of anxiety can help ease these problems.

Self-Awareness and Anxiety

Self-awareness involves noticing your own feelings and patterns. One way to build self-awareness is to pause when you feel anxious. Ask, "What is happening in my mind right now? What am I worried about?" This can reveal hidden worries. Another step is to check your body. Are your shoulders tense? Is your jaw clenched? These signals can show that anxiety is rising even before you notice it in your thoughts.

Self-awareness can help you step back and look at a problem from a distance. For example, if you see that you are worrying about being late to an appointment, you can think, "Being late might be annoying, but is it truly a disaster?" This can help you challenge the worried thought. Over time, you might find that most worries don't come true, or if they do, they are not as bad as you thought.

Learning and Changing

While anxiety can feel overwhelming, it is important to remember that people can learn ways to handle it better. Many strategies exist to manage anxious thoughts, calm the body, and make better choices in stressful times. Some include breathing exercises, problem-solving methods, or even seeking support from experts. Change may not happen overnight, but small steps can make a big difference.

It is also helpful to give credit for little wins. For example, if you normally avoid phone calls because they make you nervous, answering a call is a success. Over time, these small steps can add up. They show that anxiety does not have to control every action.

Moving Forward

Understanding anxiety is the first step in handling it. By seeing that anxiety involves both the mind and the body, people can approach it in balanced ways. By learning about common myths, recognizing thinking patterns, and seeing that anxiety comes in many forms, a person can begin to feel less alone and more in control.

Anxiety can be tricky, but there are ways to manage it that come from science and real-world practice. In the next chapters, we will explore signs and causes more closely, discuss how to handle negative thought patterns, and look at solutions that can help reduce worries. The goal is to provide practical tools that can make life easier, whether you have mild anxiety or more serious anxiety.

By reading this book, you are taking a step toward better understanding of anxiety and ways to manage it. Though it can feel tiring at times, knowledge can reduce confusion. It can also offer hope that a calmer life is possible. The rest of the chapters will share details and methods that are clear and easy to follow. There is no perfect fix, but these tips can help you lower stress, become more confident, and begin to see that anxiety does not have to rule your life.

CHAPTER 2: SIGNS AND SYMPTOMS

Anxiety can show itself in many ways. Some signs are noticed easily, like trembling or sweating. Others are hidden, like ongoing negative thoughts or a deep feeling of unease. Recognizing these signs is useful. It can guide a person to get help before the problem grows worse. This chapter will describe common signs and symptoms, how they show up in daily life, and special situations where anxiety might look different.

Physical Signs

1. **Racing Heart**: One of the most noticeable signs is a fast heartbeat. In tense situations, the heart may pound. Some people feel a flutter in their chest. This can make them think something is wrong with their body.
2. **Sweating**: Sweaty hands, damp forehead, or even soaked clothing can appear during an anxious moment. The body's temperature regulation can act up when the nervous system is on high alert.
3. **Tense Muscles**: Many people keep tension in their shoulders, neck, or jaw. They might not notice it until they feel sore or have a headache. Over time, this can lead to aches.
4. **Upset Stomach**: People with anxiety often report nausea, stomach cramps, or digestive troubles. This can happen because stress hormones change how the digestive system functions.
5. **Breathing Problems**: Some might breathe more quickly or feel short of breath. In turn, this might cause lightheadedness or a sense of choking. This can be very scary, especially if the person thinks they are in physical danger.
6. **Fatigue**: After a wave of worry, many people feel tired. The mind and body work hard when dealing with stress. This can drain energy, leading to a worn-out feeling.
7. **Shaking or Trembling**: Hands or legs might shake. This is due to the body releasing stress hormones. It might be mild or severe enough to be seen by others.

These physical signs can be confusing because they often feel like medical issues. Some people go to the emergency room thinking they have a serious heart condition. In reality, it may be a panic attack or high anxiety. That is why it's important to learn how anxiety can affect the body.

Emotional and Mental Signs

1. **Restlessness**: Feeling like you can't sit still is common. You might shift around in your seat or pace across the room.
2. **Irritability**: Anxiety can make a person short-tempered. Even small problems can feel huge. This might cause them to snap at loved ones or coworkers.
3. **Racing Thoughts**: The mind might jump from one worry to another. This can interfere with focusing on tasks. It can also keep a person awake at night.
4. **Fear of Losing Control**: Some people worry they will act strangely or lose control in public. This fear itself can feed anxiety.
5. **Sense of Doom**: A strong feeling that something terrible is about to happen. This might not be linked to any real danger, but it feels very real in the moment.
6. **Confusion**: Anxiety can cloud thinking. It might be hard to form clear thoughts or remember things.
7. **Low Mood**: Ongoing anxiety can lower a person's mood. Constant worry may result in sadness or hopelessness, though this is not always the same as depression.

Behavioral Signs

1. **Avoidance**: A common sign of anxiety is avoiding people, places, or activities. For example, someone might stop going to parties because they worry about being judged. Avoidance can lead to problems in relationships or missed chances in life.
2. **Seeking Reassurance**: Anxious individuals might frequently ask friends or family if things are okay. They want to be told that nothing bad will happen. While this might help for a short time, the relief often fades, and the anxiety returns.
3. **Perfectionism**: Some people try to lower worry by being perfect. They believe if they do everything exactly right, nothing can go wrong. This can cause high stress levels when things do not go as planned.
4. **Procrastination**: On the other hand, anxiety might cause people to put off tasks. If the thought of failing is scary, they might delay starting a project. But this can create more stress in the long run.
5. **Fidgeting**: People may tap their foot, bite their nails, or pick at their skin. These actions can be an outlet for nervous energy.

How Symptoms Show Up Over Time

Anxiety can build gradually. In the beginning, a person might have mild worries. Over time, these worries might become stronger. They might start avoiding more and more things. The body might be in a constant state of stress, leading to ongoing aches or fatigue.

Some people have waves of anxiety that come and go. They might have a period of high anxiety, then it calms down, only to return later. Others have a steady level of worry most days. The pattern can depend on life events, personal habits, and other factors.

Short-Term and Long-Term Effects

- **Short-Term**: Anxiety might help someone be cautious. But it can also trigger fight-or-flight mode, causing physical symptoms like a fast heart rate or trembling. This might affect performance on tasks that require calm thinking.
- **Long-Term**: If anxiety does not get addressed, it can cause more serious issues. The person might develop chronic tension, headaches, or digestive problems. They might lose friends if they keep avoiding social events. Their self-esteem might go down because they see themselves as unable to cope.

Special Situations and Anxiety

- **Public Speaking**: Standing in front of a crowd is a big fear for many. Signs can include sweating, shaking, or even blanking out. This is often linked to fear of judgment.
- **Medical Settings**: Some feel anxious about doctor visits, shots, or medical tests. They might worry about getting bad news. This can keep them from getting care they need.
- **Driving**: Fear of accidents or losing control while driving can be linked to anxiety. Some avoid highways or busy intersections.
- **Heights**: Many people experience intense fear at high places. It might lead to sweating, trembling, or feeling unable to move.
- **Social Gatherings**: Parties or group events can set off worries about fitting in or being laughed at. Some might fear they will say something silly.

Why Recognizing Signs Matters

Identifying signs can help someone figure out when to act. For instance, if a student knows they start to get stomach aches and headaches near exam time, they can prepare in advance. They might use stress-relieving techniques or plan their study schedule better. If someone sees that they always avoid phone calls, they can focus on practicing short calls to get used to it.

Knowing signs can also help when talking to a health professional. Instead of saying, "I just feel off," a person can say, "I notice my heart races, I feel shaky, and I avoid phone calls." This can lead to a more accurate plan to manage anxiety.

Hidden Signs

Some anxiety signs do not look like classic worry. Instead, they can look like anger, rudeness, or even lateness. A person might be late to events because they are scared they will mess up while driving. Another person might appear angry because they are trying to protect themselves from feeling too vulnerable. Understanding that anxiety can hide behind such actions can help prevent misunderstandings.

The Link with Physical Health

Anxiety can raise blood pressure, affect sleep, and strain the immune system. Lack of sleep can then cause more anxiety, forming a cycle. That is why people with chronic anxiety might get sick more often or take longer to recover from common colds. Over time, ignoring these symptoms can lead to bigger problems.

It is wise to pay attention to basic self-care. While it doesn't fix all anxiety problems, eating balanced meals, getting enough rest, and staying active can help the body handle stress better. On the other hand, skipping meals, sleeping too little, or staying indoors all day can make anxious feelings worse.

Differences Between Adults and Children

Children can show anxiety differently. They might have nightmares, refuse to go to school, or become very clingy with parents. They might also act out in anger or get upset easily. Because they have fewer words to explain their feelings, adults need to watch for changes in behavior or routine.

Teens might hide their anxiety to appear strong in front of peers. They might start missing classes, lose interest in hobbies, or begin acting in ways that appear careless. Parents or caregivers can pay attention to these warning signs. Early help can prevent bigger issues later.

When to Get Help

Some anxiety is normal. But if signs are severe, frequent, or long-lasting, it might be time to look for help. For example, if a person's worries keep them from going out, if they can't sleep most nights, or if they have ongoing panic attacks, professional care can make a difference. Reaching out to a doctor, counselor, or mental health center is a useful step.

There is no shame in needing help. Anxiety is common, and many health professionals know how to treat it. They might suggest therapy, medication, or certain exercises. The sooner someone gets help, the sooner they can see improvement.

Self-Monitoring

Self-monitoring is the act of checking your own feelings and actions. A simple method is to note in a journal whenever you feel anxious. Write down the time, place, thoughts, and how your body felt. Over a few weeks, you might see patterns. You might learn that you get more anxious in the morning or in social settings. This knowledge is powerful for making plans to ease those worries.

Some people use apps to track their mood or anxiety levels each day. They might use a scale, such as rating their anxiety from 1 to 10. Over time, the numbers can give a clear picture of progress or setbacks. This can help when deciding if certain strategies are working or if you need different methods.

Strategies to Ease Symptoms

Breathing Methods: Simple breathing techniques can calm the body. For example, you can inhale through your nose for four seconds, hold for two seconds, and exhale through your mouth for four seconds. Repeat a few times. This slows the heart rate and helps you focus on the moment.

Muscle Relaxation: Some people find it useful to tense and relax different muscle groups in the body. Start with the feet, tense them for a few seconds, then relax. Move to the calves, thighs, and so on up to the head. This can reduce overall tension.

Distraction: Doing an activity you enjoy can shift your mind away from worry. It might be a puzzle, a walk, or listening to a funny podcast. Distraction gives the anxious mind a break.

Talking to Someone: Sharing your worries with a trusted friend, family member, or expert can help lighten the burden. They might offer a new point of view or simple suggestions. Even if they don't have a solution, speaking about your feelings can bring relief.

Warning Signs of Escalation

It is important to know when anxiety is moving beyond normal levels. If your thoughts become dark or you start to think about harming yourself or others, seek help right away. If you find yourself unable to do everyday tasks because worry or panic is too strong, this signals a need for professional guidance. If panic attacks occur often and show severe physical signs, such as chest pain or trouble breathing, medical attention can rule out other causes and help manage them.

The Role of Mindset

Even though we won't go into deep detail about mindset here (since a later chapter covers it more), it is worth noting that negative thoughts can affect signs of anxiety. A simple shift from thinking, "I can't handle this," to "I'm learning to handle this," can reduce tension. Our thoughts can either increase worry or reduce it. Becoming aware of them is crucial.

CHAPTER 3: POSSIBLE CAUSES

Anxiety can come from many sources. It might be linked to brain chemistry, personal background, environment, or day-to-day habits. Some reasons are simple to see, while others are hidden. In this chapter, we will look at a range of possible causes. We will also include facts that are not always discussed, so you can understand anxiety from new angles. This can help you notice patterns in your own life and find ways to handle them.

Brain Chemistry

One reason some people feel higher levels of anxiety is linked to certain chemicals in the brain. These chemicals, sometimes called messengers, help nerve cells in the brain communicate. When there is an imbalance, the signals related to worry and fear can become too strong. This can cause the brain to stay on alert, even when threats are not real.

Some of these chemicals include serotonin, norepinephrine, and gamma-aminobutyric acid (GABA). If the levels of these chemicals are off, the mind might have a hard time calming down. While we do not always know why these chemicals become imbalanced, it can be partly due to genes or long-term stress. Modern life, with its constant news alerts and interruptions, can also keep the brain more excited than needed.

It is good to know that an imbalance does not mean a person has no control. With the right steps, the brain can become more balanced over time. These steps might include therapy, certain changes in routine, or in some cases, medication. The key idea is that anxiety is not simply a flaw. It can be partly based on biology.

Genetic and Family Factors

Family history can play a part in anxiety. Studies show that if a parent has anxiety, their child can be more at risk of having it too. This does not always mean the child will have severe worry. But it can increase the chance. Part of the reason is genes. Another part is the home environment. Children who grow up around stressed parents can learn to see the world as threatening.

Genes might make it easier for anxiety to start, but they do not decide a person's future. Some people have no family members with anxiety yet still develop it. Others have relatives with anxiety but manage to stay calm. It can help to see genes like a door that is easier to open for some. The door might open if life events push it. Still, it is possible to keep that door closed if one uses the right methods and support.

Early Life Experiences

Long before adulthood, early life events can shape a person's stress response. A child who experiences scary events at home or in the community might learn that the world is unsafe. If they also lack comfort or support, they might grow up feeling on edge.

For example, a child who faces harsh words at home might believe they are at fault for everything. This worry can extend to school or friendships, where they fear making mistakes. Another child might watch parents fight all the time, causing them to fear conflict in any form. These early experiences can store themselves in the mind and feed worry later on.

However, a rough childhood does not always lead to anxiety. Many people who had hard situations in childhood become calm and resilient adults. Supportive friends, teachers, or other mentors can help offset some of the negative patterns. The human mind is flexible and can learn better habits over time.

Life Events and Trauma

Sudden, stressful events can bring on anxiety. This might be an accident, serious illness, losing a loved one, or living through a disaster. In some cases, the memory of that event can remain strong in the mind. A person might replay it often. This leads to fear that it could happen again.

A form of anxiety known as post-traumatic stress can appear after a shocking event. Signs can include strong memories, nightmares, or a tendency to feel jumpy. Even smaller triggers, like a sound or smell that was present during the event, can cause the body's alarm system to go off. Over time, a person might try to avoid anything that reminds them of the event. This pattern can lead to more anxiety because life becomes more restricted.

Not everyone who faces a frightening event develops post-traumatic stress. Some people seem to recover faster. They might have a good network of friends, or they might have learned strong coping tools earlier in life. But if the anxiety remains, outside help can be important.

Stressful Modern Lifestyle

Many people point to the fast pace of life as a cause of ongoing worry. Emails, phone calls, social media, and work tasks can pile up. There is often a push to do more in less time. This constant "on" feeling can tax the body's stress system. The person might struggle to find quiet or time to rest. When the mind and body do not have enough rest, anxiety can build.

Some lesser-known facts show that long-term exposure to bright screens late at night might disrupt sleep. Lack of good sleep can affect hormone levels, raising anxiety risk. The body relies on deep rest to balance stress chemicals. Without it, the brain might not fully reset, leading to higher alertness during the day.

The Role of Technology

Technology is helpful in many ways, but it can also feed anxiety:

1. **Too Much Information**: Nonstop updates about global problems can make the world seem more dangerous than it is.
2. **Social Comparison**: Seeing others post only happy or perfect moments can make people feel they are not measuring up.
3. **Interrupted Focus**: Constant pings and notifications can lower attention span. The mind might lose the ability to stay calm for long.

On top of that, some studies suggest that spending too much time on screens can affect the parts of the brain that handle emotion. While technology is not always bad, it can add to anxiety if used too often or at the wrong times, such as right before bed.

Environmental Factors

Pollution or certain toxins in the environment might affect mood or the nervous system. For example, some people who live in areas with high pollution report greater stress and trouble concentrating. Mold in older buildings can also lead to physical symptoms that mimic anxiety, like dizziness or shortness of breath.

Living in noisy places might keep the brain on guard. Sirens, honking, or loud construction can keep stress hormones high. Over time, this can lead to a feeling of being on edge even when it is quiet. The mind might get used to that tense state.

Light pollution can affect the body's clock. People exposed to bright lights at night might not get good-quality sleep. Poor sleep is strongly linked to anxiety. Finding ways to reduce unwanted noise and light at home can help.

Social Pressures

People often face pressure to fit in, do well in school or work, and meet family expectations. Over time, these pressures can push a person's stress levels higher. Some might worry they will disappoint others if they do not meet certain standards. This can cause them to try too hard or become fearful of mistakes.

In school settings, big exams or competition can lead to ongoing worry. In the workplace, heavy workloads or fear of losing a job can keep stress at a high level. If someone does not have healthy ways to cope or share these concerns, anxiety can worsen.

There is also the matter of social standing. Some people fear not being liked or being misunderstood. They might scan every interaction for signs that others are judging them. This fear can drain mental energy, leading to more worry.

Hormonal Imbalances

Hormones do many jobs in the body. When hormones shift too much or too fast, anxiety can go up. For instance, if certain stress hormones like cortisol remain high for a long time, it can create ongoing tension. Some people have overactive thyroid glands, which can cause a racing heart or panic feelings.

Certain times of life, such as puberty, pregnancy, or menopause, involve big hormonal shifts. These periods can be tough because the body is changing. If the person is already prone to worry, these shifts might make things worse for a while. Checking for hormonal issues with a doctor can sometimes explain sudden anxiety spikes.

Nutritional Factors

Not many people think of nutrition when they feel anxious, but what we eat has an effect on the mind. For example, low levels of vitamin B12 or vitamin D can lead to anxiety symptoms. A body that lacks these vitamins might have trouble regulating mood.

Caffeine is another factor. A morning cup of coffee can give a boost, but too much caffeine during the day can cause jittery feelings. It might also disturb sleep if taken late in the day, which can then raise anxiety levels the next day. Sugar highs and crashes can also influence how the brain feels. Some people find that cutting back on sugary foods helps them feel more stable.

A healthy diet, filled with whole foods, fruits, vegetables, and enough protein, can help the brain work at its best. While diet alone may not solve all anxiety problems, it is a piece of the puzzle that should not be ignored.

Substances and Medication Side Effects

Some medications can cause anxiety as a side effect. This can include certain asthma medicines, steroids, or pills for attention problems. If someone suddenly notices more worry after starting a new medication, it is wise to talk to a doctor.

Alcohol or drug use can also play a part. Some people drink or use other substances to calm nerves. But this often causes a bounce-back effect. Once the substance wears off, anxiety can come back stronger. Over time, the body might rely on the substance, creating a cycle that is hard to break.

Even nicotine can raise the heart rate and blood pressure, which might increase anxious feelings. Cutting out certain substances, under proper guidance, may lower anxiety.

Personality Traits

Some personality styles lean more toward being tense or worried. For instance, people who like everything planned out might feel uneasy when there is uncertainty. While being organized can be useful, if it becomes extreme, the person might panic if things do not go as expected.

Another personality trait is high sensitivity. A sensitive person might feel emotions more deeply. Loud noises, chaotic places, or arguments might affect them strongly, raising their anxiety. This is not a bad trait, but it means they might need extra methods to lower stress.

The Gut-Brain Connection

A lesser-known area involves the gut and its link to the brain. Scientists have found that bacteria in the digestive system can affect mood and anxiety. If the mix of bacteria is off, it might change the way the body produces certain chemicals that calm the mind.

Some research shows that adding certain fermented foods, rich in good bacteria, may help the brain. This does not mean it cures all anxiety, but it can be a small factor that contributes to better emotional balance. On the other hand, a diet high in processed foods might harm the gut's balance, possibly affecting mood.

Weather and Seasons

Some people notice their anxiety rises during certain seasons. This can be due to changes in sunlight or lower temperatures. It can also be linked to how much time is spent indoors versus outside. Less time in natural light might reduce vitamin D levels, which can affect mood.

Sudden weather shifts, like storms or high humidity, can also cause discomfort that might trigger anxiety in sensitive individuals. They might feel the pressure changes in their body. While this does not affect everyone, it is an interesting factor for those who notice anxiety on rainy or gloomy days.

Loneliness and Isolation

Humans are social by nature. When a person feels isolated or lonely, it can boost negative thoughts. Without close connections, a small worry might grow bigger in the mind because there is no one around to provide balance or support.

Modern living can make loneliness more common. People might move away from family for work, or they might rely on social media instead of face-to-face time. While online contact can help, it often does not replace real companionship. Over time, this gap can feed anxiety, especially if the person feels they have no one to talk to about their worries.

Hidden Health Conditions

Sometimes anxiety is a sign that something else is happening in the body. Thyroid disorders, heart issues, or breathing problems might show themselves through worry or panic feelings. Vitamin or mineral deficiencies can also set off anxious moods.

That is why it can be helpful to rule out hidden health problems if anxiety appears suddenly or feels extreme. Seeing a medical professional can make sure there is no underlying issue. If a problem is found, treating it might reduce the anxiety.

Learning Anxiety from Others

In families or groups of friends, people can pick up anxious habits. For example, if parents are always worried about money, a child might grow up feeling that money is always a threat. If friends constantly talk about worst-case scenarios, a person might start to do the same. Over time, these learned thoughts can become normal.

Once the person notices this pattern, they can start to adopt different ways of thinking. They might read self-help books or talk to people who manage stress better. This can show them that not everyone reacts to events with worry. Learning new responses can reduce anxiety that was picked up from others.

Cumulative Effect

Sometimes, there is not one big cause of anxiety but rather a buildup of small issues. A person might have a mild tendency to worry, come from a family with some anxiety, then add in a busy job, plus a bit of poor diet. Put it all together, and the level of anxiety can get high.

This is why it is wise to look at your life as a whole. Maybe none of the factors alone seem big, but combined, they form a wave of stress. Addressing them one by one can lower that stress. For example, a small improvement in diet, a bit of daily quiet time, and a reduction in screen exposure might work together to reduce overall worry.

Why Causes Matter

Learning about the possible causes of anxiety helps you understand it is not random or entirely out of your control. You might identify specific factors in your own life. This can lead to targeted steps. For example, if you notice caffeine makes you jittery, you can reduce it. If you realize bright lights in your bedroom keep you from good sleep, you can try blackout curtains or turn off devices earlier in the evening.

Knowing the causes can also reduce shame. Some people think anxiety means they are weak. But often, it is a response to certain triggers or physical issues. Recognizing these triggers can help a person feel more at peace, because they see the logical reasons behind their feelings.

Action Steps to Manage Causes

1. **Medical Checkup**: If anxiety is high, consider seeing a doctor. They can test for thyroid problems or nutrient gaps.
2. **Review Medications**: If you have recently started a new medication, ask the doctor if anxiety might be a side effect.
3. **Consider the Gut**: If you suspect your digestion might affect your mood, talk to a nutrition specialist. Simple diet changes or probiotic-rich foods might help.
4. **Limit Screen Time**: Try cutting down on device use, especially at night. This can help regulate sleep and reduce mental overload.
5. **Balance Caffeine**: If you love coffee, note how you feel after drinking it. See if stopping earlier in the day helps.
6. **Seek Support**: If big life events are causing worry, it might help to talk with a friend, counselor, or support group.
7. **Reduce Noise and Light**: If possible, use earplugs or noise-blocking curtains to create a calmer space. Blackout curtains can help sleep.
8. **Check Work-Life Balance**: If you are constantly doing tasks or thinking about them, set specific times to rest or focus on a hobby.

Putting It All Together

Anxiety does not come from one cause alone. It can arise from genes, early life, environment, daily habits, or health factors. Recognizing the mix of causes that apply to you can lead to better solutions. If you ignore these causes, anxiety can remain or even grow. But if you face them, you can lower stress in small but real ways.

This chapter highlights many possible triggers that may not be commonly discussed, such as gut health or small toxins in the environment. By paying attention to these factors, you can piece together clues about your own anxiety. You might find it useful to keep track of your diet, your environment, and your daily stress levels. Over time, patterns may appear that you can address with targeted steps.

CHAPTER 4: NEGATIVE THINKING PATTERNS

An anxious mind often involves negative thought patterns. These are habits of thinking that can increase worry or create false beliefs about life. By spotting and changing these thought patterns, a person can lower anxiety and see events in a more realistic way. In this chapter, we will explore how negative thinking works, how it harms mental health, and how to break free from it. We will also include some useful tips that are not always found in regular guides.

What Are Negative Thinking Patterns?

Negative thinking patterns are automatic ways the mind can twist reality. The person might expect terrible outcomes or only focus on bad details. The main issue is that these patterns often run in the background, so the person might not notice them. They might think these thoughts are normal. But when the mind defaults to negative views, it can cause more anxiety than necessary.

For instance, you might see a small problem and assume it signals a chain of disasters. Or you might make one mistake and conclude you are a failure. Over time, these negative thoughts build up, making you feel nervous or upset even when there is no serious problem.

Common Negative Thought Patterns

1. **All-or-Nothing Thinking**: Seeing things in extreme terms, such as a performance being perfect or worthless. There is no middle ground. For example, if you get one question wrong on a test, you might see it as a total failure, ignoring the many questions you got right.
2. **Overgeneralizing**: Taking one event and turning it into a broad rule about life. For instance, if you once missed a job opportunity, you might think you will always fail at finding work. This can push you to feel hopeless about future efforts.
3. **Mental Filter**: Focusing on only the bad parts of a situation and ignoring the good. Suppose you do well on a project, but you highlight one small flaw in it. You keep replaying that flaw, making you feel like the project was a disaster.

4. **Discounting Positives**: You might see your successes but dismiss them as luck or not a big deal. This can keep you stuck in a mindset where nothing positive counts.
5. **Jumping to Conclusions**: Making negative guesses without real proof. This often involves two types:
    - **Mind Reading**: You assume you know what others are thinking, usually something bad about you.
    - **Fortune Telling**: You predict the future will be negative or that things will go wrong, even if there is no proof.
6. **Catastrophizing**: Expecting the worst possible outcome, even for minor events. If you get a small headache, you might believe it is a serious illness. This pattern can raise anxiety levels quickly.
7. **Emotional Reasoning**: Believing that your feelings define reality. For instance, "I feel scared, so the situation must be dangerous." Your feelings can be real, but they are not always accurate about how risky a situation is.
8. **Labeling**: Putting a harsh label on yourself or someone else based on one event. For example, calling yourself a "loser" because you failed one test. These labels can be hard to remove once you start using them.
9. **Should Statements**: Telling yourself you "should" or "must" do something in a certain way. This can lead to guilt or shame if you cannot meet those strict standards.

How Negative Thinking Fuels Anxiety

When negative thoughts appear, they often trigger a physical stress response. The body can release stress hormones, making your heart beat faster or your muscles tense. This only adds to the sense that something is wrong. If this cycle continues, it can lead to frequent anxiety or panic. It becomes a loop: negative thought → body reacts → mind thinks it must be true → more worry.

Additionally, these thoughts can stop a person from seeing positive options. If you believe you will fail, you might not try new things. If you think everyone dislikes you, you might avoid social contacts. This can trap you in situations where anxiety grows because you never learn a different viewpoint.

Why We Develop Negative Patterns

Negative thinking patterns often start in childhood or after repeated stress. A child who is punished harshly for small mistakes may learn all-or-nothing thinking. A teen who experiences rejection might decide that they are unlikable. Over time, the mind uses these shortcuts to make sense of the world.

Sometimes, society or media might teach us certain fears. Constant bad news can push a person to expect the worst. Another reason is that worrying can feel like a form of protection. People think if they worry enough, they can prepare for bad outcomes. But usually, it just increases stress without truly preventing problems.

Spotting Negative Thoughts

A first step to breaking negative patterns is to notice them. Because these thoughts are often quick and automatic, it helps to pause and question what the mind is saying. For example, if you are feeling a rush of anxiety about an event, ask yourself, "What am I thinking right now?" Write it down. You might see a sentence like, "I know I will mess this up."

Next, ask if this statement is fact or just a guess. You might see you have no real proof that you will mess up. In fact, you might have done well in similar situations. By labeling the thought as negative rather than truth, you create space to adjust it.

Replacing Negative Thoughts

1. **Examine Evidence**: Treat your thought like a claim in an argument. Gather proof for and against it. Often, you will see the negative thought is not fully supported by facts.
2. **Use Balanced Statements**: Instead of saying, "I will fail for sure," say, "I have a chance to do well, and if I make mistakes, I can learn from them." This does not paint a picture of guaranteed success, but it also does not assume disaster.

3. **Positive Self-Talk**: Some people find it helpful to have short phrases ready, such as "I can handle this," or "I have dealt with challenges before." Repeating these can calm the anxious mind.
4. **Look for Exceptions**: If you think, "I always mess up," try to find times you succeeded. This stops the mind from ignoring positive evidence.
5. **Set Realistic Goals**: If you think, "I must never make a mistake," remind yourself that mistakes are part of life. Aim to do your best, not to be perfect.

Handling Thoughts in Real Time

It can be tough to catch negative thoughts in the middle of daily tasks. A helpful trick is to use a quick mental signal, like saying "Stop" to yourself when you notice a negative spiral. Then, shift your focus to something more grounded, like the sensation of your feet on the floor or the sounds around you. This moment of pause can break the chain of anxious thinking.

Another idea is to assign a short period for worrying. For example, set aside 10 minutes in the evening to sit down and write your worries. If a worry pops up during the day, tell yourself you will look at it in the "worry period." This can reduce the constant chatter of anxious thoughts. When the scheduled time arrives, you might find some worries already feel less serious.

Hidden Traps in Negative Thinking

Sometimes, negative thinking patterns disguise themselves as being practical. For example, you might say, "I'm just being realistic." But if you always imagine the worst outcome, that is not simply realistic. Another trap is thinking that negative thoughts push you to work harder. While a bit of caution can motivate, harsh thoughts often cause burnout or avoidance.

Also, negative patterns can spread into many areas of life. You might start with one fear about your health. Then it expands to worry about your relationships, your job, or the future. Being aware of how these thoughts spread can help you catch them sooner.

Advanced Tips for Breaking Negative Patterns

- **Name the Voice**: Give your negative inner voice a nickname. This might sound silly, but it helps you separate the negative talk from your true self. When it appears, you can say, "Oh, that's just [nickname], giving the same old story."
- **Use Humor**: Gently making fun of extreme thoughts can cut their power. For example, if you catch yourself thinking, "Everything will collapse," you could picture a silly cartoon scene. This approach helps you see the thought as exaggerated.
- **Thought Swapping**: Have a set of realistic but calming thoughts ready in a list or on your phone. When you spot a negative thought, replace it with one from the list. This trains the mind to shift direction.
- **Group Support**: Sometimes talking to others who have similar worries helps you see your thoughts are not unique. Hearing how they replace negative thoughts can give you fresh ideas.
- **Small Experiments**: If your negative thought is, "I can't handle going out," plan a small outing and see if that is true. Real-life success can help break the belief. Even if it feels scary, the actual experience might show you are stronger than you thought.

Impact on Confidence

When negative thoughts run free, they can damage self-confidence. You might feel worthless or see yourself as a problem. Over time, this can lead to a loss of motivation. You may not try new things because you believe you will fail. Breaking negative thinking patterns can rebuild confidence. As you allow for the idea that you can do okay or even well, you open paths to new experiences.

Confidence grows when you test your fears in small steps and see that outcomes are not as bad as you expected. Each success, however small, challenges the negative voice in your head. Over time, these successes can stack up, giving you a new track record that you can rely on.

Effects on Relationships

Negative thinking does not just affect your inner world. It also impacts how you see and treat others. If you assume friends are judging you, you might act distant or defensive. If you expect conflict, you might avoid talking about important topics. These habits can strain friendships or family ties.

By noticing your thought patterns about others, you can become fairer and calmer in your interactions. For example, instead of thinking, "They didn't text me back because they hate me," consider simpler reasons, like they might be busy. This can stop you from getting upset or pulling away when it is not really needed.

Helping Others with Negative Thinking

Sometimes, you will see negative patterns in people you care about. While you cannot force them to change their mindset, you can suggest ways to question their thoughts. Share simple techniques, like writing down worries or looking for evidence. Offer a listening ear without judging. By being supportive, you might help them step back from destructive thinking.

On the other hand, do not feel you must fix everyone's negative thoughts. If the issue is deep, encourage them to seek professional help. You can be there for them, but they might need tools that only a counselor or mental health professional can provide.

Deeper Connection to Anxiety

Many of the worries that feed anxiety come from these thinking patterns. A small moment of concern can snowball into a huge problem in the mind. If you reduce negative patterns, you remove a major source of fuel for anxiety. While you cannot control every random thought, you can shape how you respond.

For instance, if you catch yourself catastrophizing about being late, you can challenge that thought. Ask, "Will being late once ruin my entire life?" The realistic answer might be that it is only a slight problem, and you can manage. This calmer view helps your body relax, lowering the anxious response.

Practical Exercises

1. **Daily Thought Check**: Once or twice a day, write down any strong worries you had, what triggered them, and what negative pattern might have been at play. Then rewrite a balanced thought.
2. **Visualize a Positive Outcome**: If you often predict the worst, take a moment to picture a better scenario. This is not about fooling yourself but giving your mind the chance to see another path.
3. **Gratitude List**: Each day, list a few things that went well or that you appreciate. This helps balance the mind if it leans toward negative details.
4. **Neutral Observation**: When you feel negative thoughts, pretend you are a neutral reporter. Describe the situation without adding words like "terrible" or "awful." This can help you see events without the emotional weight.

Checking for Progress

Over time, you can track if these methods are reducing negative thoughts. Maybe you notice you no longer call yourself harsh names. Or you might see you handle small setbacks without spiraling. Recognizing progress is important. It encourages you to keep up the effort.

However, do not expect a quick fix. Negative patterns built up over years often take time to change. The mind might slip back now and then. If that happens, remind yourself it is part of the process. Return to the methods that worked before.

When More Help Is Needed

If negative thoughts are so strong that they lead to constant anxiety, it might be good to seek professional input. A therapist or counselor can guide you in spotting thoughts you miss or provide structured plans to reshape them. Sometimes group therapy can help, as listening to others' stories reveals how common these patterns are.

In more severe cases, medication could be an option. But even with medication, learning to handle negative thoughts remains useful. Medication might calm the body's stress response, but the thought habits could still be there if you do not work on them.

Connecting with Other Techniques

Breaking negative thought patterns often goes with other anxiety-reducing methods. For example, breathing exercises can help calm you enough so you can spot your thoughts more clearly. Good sleep, healthy eating, and regular physical activity can also lower overall stress, giving you more mental energy to fight unhelpful beliefs.

Mindful practices, where you pay attention to the present without judging it, can also help. By staying in the present, you reduce the mind's urge to jump to scary future scenarios or replay past mistakes.

Moving Forward

Negative thinking patterns can trap a person in a cycle of anxiety. These patterns may come from childhood, society, or simple habits. Yet they can be changed with practice. By catching negative thoughts, questioning them, and replacing them with balanced views, you can greatly reduce the strain they cause.

In the next chapters, we will continue exploring ways to handle anxiety from different angles. We will look at stress management, self-talk, and other tools that add to your mental health. Each chapter will build on what we have covered so far, giving you a broad set of methods to try. As you keep applying these tips, you might find that life feels less scary, and your mind feels calmer. This can open doors to new experiences and better daily satisfaction.

Keep in mind that negative thinking does not mean you are doomed. It is a habit that can be changed over time. By taking small steps, you lay a foundation for a different approach to challenges. Whether you use thought checks, balanced statements, or group support, each step helps reshape how you see yourself and the world. Over time, you can find that anxiety loses some of its power, allowing you to move through your days with more calm and certainty.

CHAPTER 5: SELF-TALK

Self-talk means the running words in your head. It is the inner dialogue you have with yourself throughout the day. Often, people do not notice this chatter. It can be either supportive or harsh. When it is harsh, it can add to anxiety and low mood. When it is supportive, it can bring calmness and hope. In this chapter, we will explore how self-talk forms, why it matters for mental health, and how to change it so it helps rather than harms. We will also look at clear tips that people can use right away.

What Is Self-Talk?

Self-talk is the commentary that plays in a person's mind. It happens when you wake up thinking, "I have a busy day," or when you drop something and say to yourself, "I'm so clumsy." This voice is a pattern shaped by your background, your beliefs, and the events you have been through. At times, it can be positive. For example, "I will do my best on this test." Other times, it can be negative. For example, "I know I'm going to fail."

Because self-talk is so constant, it can shape how you feel and act without you realizing it. If you tell yourself that you are worthless many times a day, you might start to feel sad or anxious, even if there is no clear reason for it. On the other hand, if your inner voice is encouraging, you might face challenges with more strength.

Why Self-Talk Affects Anxiety

Anxiety can rise or fall depending on your thoughts. If your inner voice leans toward worry, it can feed anxiety in many ways:

1. **Exaggerating Dangers**: Saying things to yourself like, "Everything is going wrong," can make a small problem seem like a huge threat.
2. **Constant Self-Blame**: Telling yourself you are lazy or foolish can build shame. That shame often leads to more worry about how others see you.

3. **Predicting Failure**: Repeating thoughts such as, "I won't be able to handle it," can stop you from trying new things. This leads to missed chances and more fear of the unknown.
4. **Undermining Confidence**: If you keep telling yourself that you are weak, you might hesitate in moments that need calm focus. Then you might fail not because you cannot do it, but because you did not give yourself a fair chance.

Self-talk can be subtle. You might not say "I'm worthless" directly, but you might think, "I never do anything right," or "My opinion does not matter." Over time, these beliefs collect in the mind, adding tension and worry.

Where Harsh Self-Talk Comes From

Self-talk patterns often form early in life. If you heard negative remarks from parents, teachers, or friends, you might begin repeating those remarks in your own mind. For instance, if a parent always said, "You're so lazy," the child might take on that label. Once grown, the child-turned-adult could still think, "I'm lazy," even if that is not true at all.

Society also influences self-talk. Advertisements might imply you are not good-looking enough unless you buy a certain product. Social media could make you think you are not successful if you do not match the images you see. These outside voices can seep into your inner voice.

Stressful events can magnify negative self-talk as well. If something tragic happens, you might conclude you deserved it, or you were at fault. This can lead to self-blame that becomes a habit. Recognizing these roots can help you understand why certain messages keep playing in your head.

The Effects of Supportive Self-Talk

On the positive side, supportive self-talk can do wonders:

1. **Motivation**: Telling yourself, "I'm improving bit by bit," can push you to keep trying.
2. **Calming**: Reassuring words, like, "I can handle this," can lower tension in anxious moments.

3. **Building Confidence**: Recognizing your own efforts leads you to trust your skills. Over time, this can help you try new things without fear.
4. **Better Mood**: Supportive self-talk can reduce sadness or anger, allowing you to focus on solutions instead of getting stuck in blame.

It is important to note that supportive self-talk does not mean lying to yourself. It is not about saying, "I will never have problems." Rather, it is about a balanced view. For instance, "I'm having a tough day, but I have managed tough days before."

Recognizing Your Inner Voice

Many people do not pay attention to their self-talk. It happens in the background like background noise. To notice it, you can try the following:

1. **Writing Thoughts**: Set aside a short time each day to write down whatever is running through your mind. Do not worry about neatness or grammar. Just record the words and see if they are positive, negative, or neutral.
2. **Using a Timer**: Every few hours, set a reminder on your phone. When it goes off, quickly note the main thoughts you had in the last five minutes.
3. **Listening for Repeated Phrases**: Notice if certain lines repeat, like "I'm not smart enough," or "No one cares what I think." These are clues to your self-talk style.
4. **Talking Out Loud**: Sometimes speaking your thoughts out loud can highlight whether they sound mean or kind.

At first, you might be surprised by how often you criticize yourself in your mind. Do not panic if you discover many negative lines. Spotting them is a good first step toward change.

Changing the Inner Script

Once you see a pattern of harsh self-talk, you can work on shifting it. This is not about going from "I'm a total failure" to "I'm the best person in the world." It is about moving from extreme negativity to balanced thinking.

1. **Challenge the Thought**: When you hear a harsh thought, ask yourself if it is accurate. Is there real evidence? Often, you will find it is an assumption or an exaggeration.
2. **Replace It with a Balanced Statement**: For example, if the negative thought is, "I always mess up," you might replace it with, "I have messed up before, but I've also done okay many times."
3. **Use a Friend Test**: If a friend were saying this about themselves, what would you tell them? Usually, we are kinder to friends than to ourselves. Apply that same kindness to your own mind.
4. **Keep It Short**: Have a few short, helpful phrases ready. For instance:
   - "I can take small steps."
   - "I am making progress."
   - "One mistake does not define me."
   - "I'm learning how to cope."
5. **Practice**: Each time you notice harsh self-talk, do your best to replace it. This might feel strange at first, but over time, it becomes more natural.

Avoiding the Trap of False Positivity

Some people swing to the other extreme, trying to force only cheerful thoughts. This can be confusing because it can lead to ignoring real problems. The goal is not to pretend everything is perfect. It is to look at facts in a balanced way. If you feel anxious about a work project, it might be because there are real tasks to do. The balanced thought is, "I have a lot to do, but I have a plan. I can handle it step by step."

Ignoring real concerns can cause them to grow bigger. Healthy self-talk accepts problems but does not assume they are the end of the world. It finds a middle path between extreme negativity and fake positivity.

Self-Talk in Specific Situations

1. **Before Stressful Events**: If you have to speak in front of people, your mind might jump to, "I will forget my words." A healthier line would be, "I might feel nervous, but I have practiced. I can do my best." This small shift can lower the threat level in your mind.

2. **After Mistakes**: When you make a mistake, harsh self-talk might say, "I'm such a loser." A kinder view is, "I made an error, but I can fix it or learn from it next time."
3. **During Conflict**: If you argue with someone, you might think, "They hate me." A calmer thought might be, "We had a disagreement, but that does not mean they hate me. We can find a solution if we talk calmly."

By choosing a different inner dialogue, you reduce the tension in your body and mind. This does not fix everything instantly, but it gives you more room to take good actions.

The Role of Self-Compassion

Self-compassion is about treating yourself kindly, especially in moments of failure or pain. Many people feel it is easy to be kind to others but hard to be kind to themselves. This gap can keep you stuck in harsh self-talk. If you approach yourself with understanding instead of scolding, you can reduce anxiety. Ask yourself:

- "How would I support a friend going through this?"
- "Is it possible I am being too hard on myself?"

Compassion does not mean letting yourself off the hook for bad choices. It simply means you are not adding extra pain through insults or guilt. You can accept that you made a mistake while still choosing to do better next time.

Tools and Exercises for Better Self-Talk

1. **Mirror Exercise**: Stand in front of a mirror and say one kind statement about yourself. This might feel odd at first, but it helps you become aware of your tone.
2. **Thought Cards**: Write short supportive lines on small cards. Keep them in your wallet or phone. When you notice harsh thoughts, read your helpful lines.
3. **Recording Progress**: Each day, note one thing you did that you are proud of, even if it is small. This builds evidence for positive self-talk.

4. **Name the Harsh Voice**: Give the harsh inner voice a silly name. Then, when it speaks up, you can mentally say, "Oh, that's just that voice again. I don't have to listen."
5. **Question Yourself**: If you think, "I can't do it," ask "What if I can do a part of it? Or get help if I need it?" This opens doors rather than shutting them.

Group Support and Self-Talk

Talking with others can also help. Sometimes we are so used to our own minds that we cannot see how negative we sound. If a friend or a counselor hears you say, "I'll never succeed," they can point out that this might not be true. They can remind you of times you did succeed. Joining a support group where people share tips about handling stress can also be helpful. Hearing other people's self-talk stories might show you that you are not the only one who struggles with a critical mind.

Children and Self-Talk

Children often pick up self-talk from adults around them. If a parent or teacher constantly says, "I'm no good at anything," the child may repeat that pattern. Helping children learn supportive self-talk early can protect them from years of anxiety. If a child gets frustrated with homework and says, "I can't do this," a helpful reply might be, "You're finding it hard right now, but let's see which part you can handle. We can work on it step by step." Over time, this can shape a healthy inner voice for the child as they grow.

When Self-Talk Becomes Dangerous

Sometimes, harsh self-talk can become extremely negative. It may say things like, "I don't deserve to be happy," or "I am a burden." This is serious because it can lead to harmful thoughts or actions. If you or someone you know has such thoughts, it is crucial to reach out to a mental health professional as soon as possible. These feelings can be improved with the right care, but they need urgent attention.

Avoiding Self-Talk Pitfalls

As you work on self-talk, watch out for subtle traps:

1. **Comparisons**: You might still compare yourself to others: "I am doing better, but I'm not as good as my friend." This can bring back negative thoughts. Stick to your own progress.
2. **Perfection**: You might expect that your self-talk must be positive all the time. That is not realistic. Occasionally you will have negative thoughts. The goal is to notice them and return to balance, not to be perfect.
3. **Expecting Instant Results**: Shifting self-talk is a gradual process. You may feel a slight lift quickly, but deep change usually needs practice.
4. **Using Self-Talk as a Shield**: Some people might try to cover up problems with over-the-top statements like, "I am the greatest ever." This can hide real fears that need attention. Balanced self-talk addresses fear in a calm way rather than ignoring it.

Tracking Improvements

Consider keeping a small chart or journal to track your progress each day or week. Note when you used harsh self-talk and how you replaced it. Notice if your anxiety levels dropped after you switched to a more caring stance. Over a few weeks, you might see patterns, such as:

- You have more negative thoughts when you are tired.
- You have less harsh self-talk after talking with supportive friends.
- You replace negative thoughts more easily now than at the start.

Seeing these improvements can encourage you to keep going.

Linking Self-Talk with Other Skills

Better self-talk goes well with other anxiety-reducing steps, such as breathing methods, physical activity, or good sleep habits. For example, if you combine supportive self-talk with short relaxation breaks, you might notice a strong drop in stress. Each technique can make the others stronger.

If you are already working with a counselor, you can share your self-talk progress with them. They may have extra tips to help you deal with stubborn negative lines. The more tools you gather, the easier it can be to face big life challenges.

Self-Talk in the Long Run

Changing self-talk is not a quick fix. It is a life habit. Over time, you might catch yourself automatically choosing kinder words. This does not mean you will never think negative thoughts. Everyone has rough days or moments of doubt. But the difference is that you will not stay stuck there. You will have the skill to shift your mindset and find calmness again.

When supportive self-talk becomes normal, it can help you face many areas of life. You might speak up more in group settings because your mind no longer tells you, "No one cares what you have to say." You might try new hobbies because you do not fear failure so much. You might even feel more compassion for others because you understand how big a difference simple encouraging words can make.

Putting It All Together

Self-talk is a powerful force that can either boost or drag you down. By paying attention, you can find patterns in your mind's chatter. If it is negative, you can shift it to balanced words that recognize both challenges and strengths. Over time, this can greatly reduce anxiety and open the door to healthier thinking. Even if you have long-standing harsh thoughts, you can learn to replace them with lines that help you do better.

In the next chapter, we will explore how to handle stress. Anxiety often grows when stress is high, and learning to manage stress can prevent it from overwhelming you. Self-talk and stress management work together to provide a solid base for mental health. By working on both, you can grow stronger from the inside out. Self-talk is one piece of the bigger picture. Use it wisely, and you will find it can be a steady guide in stressful or uncertain times.

CHAPTER 6: STRESS MANAGEMENT

Stress is a part of everyday life. It shows up when we face deadlines, arguments, or big changes. A little stress can drive us to take action. But too much stress can overload the body and mind, leading to anxiety, anger, or sickness. In this chapter, we will look at how stress forms, how it affects the body, and ways to keep it under control. We will also add some helpful ideas that go beyond simple tips, giving you new ways to see and handle your stress.

What Causes Stress?

Stress can come from various places:

1. **Work or School**: Deadlines, tests, or a heavy workload can create ongoing pressure.
2. **Relationships**: Conflict with friends, family, or coworkers can lead to emotional strain.
3. **Life Changes**: Moving to a new place, losing a job, or even positive changes like having a baby can increase stress.
4. **Health Problems**: Chronic pain or concerns about illness can make day-to-day life feel uncertain.
5. **Daily Hassles**: Traffic jams, long lines, or sudden errands can pile up and push stress to a higher level.

Sometimes stress builds slowly, like water filling a container. One drop is not a big deal, but over time, the container might overflow. Recognizing this buildup is important so you can act before it becomes overwhelming.

The Stress Response in the Body

When you face stress, your body releases hormones such as adrenaline and cortisol. These chemicals speed up your heart rate and tighten your muscles. This is a natural process that prepares you to handle challenges. Once the challenge passes, the body is supposed to reset. However, if stress stays high for a long time, the body might remain tense. This can lead to:

- Ongoing fatigue

- Weakened immune system
- Trouble sleeping
- Digestive issues
- Tension headaches or muscle pain

In addition, long-term stress can affect mood. It can push a person toward anxiety or sadness. That is why stress management is a key part of mental health. If you lower stress, you often lower anxiety too.

Stress vs. Anxiety

Stress is often linked to a clear cause. For example, you have a big assignment due tomorrow, and you feel under pressure. Once you finish the assignment, stress should lessen. Anxiety, on the other hand, can linger even when the original cause is gone or unclear. You might feel uneasy all day, without knowing exactly why.

However, stress can spill over into anxiety if it stays high. The body might learn to stay in an alert state, scanning for problems. If there is always one new issue after another, the mind does not get a break. This can lead to chronic anxiety. Recognizing when stress is turning into anxiety can help you step in with solutions.

Identifying Your Stress Signs

People show stress in different ways. Some might get headaches; others might become irritable or lose their appetite. Common signs include:

1. **Physical Tension**: Tight shoulders, clenched jaw, or back pain.
2. **Rapid Breathing**: Feeling like you cannot catch your breath.
3. **Racing Thoughts**: Finding it hard to focus because worries jump around in your mind.
4. **Change in Sleep**: Sleeping too much or too little.
5. **Upset Stomach**: Nausea, stomach pains, or bowel issues.

Learning your personal signs can help you spot when you are nearing your limit. You can then use coping methods rather than waiting until you feel completely overwhelmed.

Setting Boundaries

One main method to lower stress is setting clear boundaries. This can mean saying "no" to extra tasks when you are already busy. It might involve taking breaks from social media if it is causing you stress. Or it can mean telling people what times you are not available to talk about work.

Boundaries might be hard to set if you worry about letting people down. But without them, you risk burning out. It is okay to protect your time and energy. In fact, having good boundaries can make you more helpful in the long run because you are not running on empty.

Time Management

Many people feel stressed because they have a lot to do but not enough time. You can reduce this by using some time management basics:

1. **Plan Your Day**: Write down what you need to do. Put the most urgent or important tasks first.
2. **Break Tasks Down**: A big project can feel less scary if you turn it into smaller steps.
3. **Use a Timer**: Work in focused sessions, then take short breaks. This method helps prevent burnout.
4. **Cut Down Distractions**: Close apps or tabs you do not need. Decide when you will check messages rather than checking every few minutes.

Finding a system that fits your style can reduce the feeling of being rushed. When you can see progress, stress often goes down. It also gives you a sense of control, which helps keep anxiety away.

Relaxation Techniques

Relaxation methods are physical or mental exercises that lower tension. Here are some:

1. **Deep Breathing**: Inhale slowly through your nose, count to four, hold for a second or two, then exhale through your mouth for a count of four. Repeat a few times. This signals your body to calm down.

2. **Progressive Muscle Relaxation**: Tense one muscle group at a time (like your fists), hold for five seconds, then release. Move through different areas of your body.
3. **Visualization**: Picture a calm place, like a quiet park. Focus on details such as the colors, sounds, or smells. This can trick your brain into reducing stress responses.
4. **Mindful Observation**: Pick an object around you (like a pen). Examine it for a minute, noticing its texture, color, and shape. This helps draw attention away from racing thoughts.

These might sound simple, but they can cause a real drop in stress when practiced regularly. Some people use an app or guided audio to walk them through these steps.

Physical Activity and Stress

Physical activity is a known stress reliever. It can be as basic as a short walk or a set of stretches. When you move, your body releases chemicals that help you feel better. It also helps relax tense muscles. You do not need a long or intense workout. Even 10 or 15 minutes can be enough to shift your mood.

Try different forms of exercise to see what you enjoy. It might be dancing, gentle yoga stretches, biking, or playing a sport. The key is to find something that feels fun or at least satisfying. If you hate running, do not force yourself to run. Pick an activity that you can do often without dread.

Nutrition and Stress

Stress can lead to mindless eating, such as grabbing sugary snacks or drinks. While these might give a quick boost, they often lead to a crash later. This crash can feel like more stress. Instead, aim for balanced meals with protein, complex carbs, fruits, and vegetables. Drinking enough water also helps keep your mind clear.

Small changes can make a difference. For example, swapping soda for water, or adding an extra serving of vegetables, can help your body handle stress. Some people also find herbal teas soothing. The idea is not to follow a strict diet, but to choose foods that give you steady energy.

Sleep and Stress

Lack of sleep is a big source of stress. When the body does not get enough rest, it is more sensitive to daily problems. You might find small things, like a slow computer, making you angry or worried. Over time, sleep debt can lead to health issues and increased anxiety.

To improve sleep:

1. **Avoid Bright Screens Before Bed**: The light from phones or TVs can confuse your body's internal clock.
2. **Keep a Cool, Dark Space**: A comfortable environment supports deep sleep.
3. **Reduce Noise**: Use earplugs or a fan to mask sudden sounds.
4. **Have a Wind-Down Routine**: For example, read a simple book or do gentle stretches.
5. **Limit Caffeine Late in the Day**: Caffeine can last in your system for hours, messing with your ability to fall asleep.

With better sleep, your mind is more resilient. You can tackle daily stress without feeling drained.

Social Support

People often forget that sharing stress with someone you trust can lower its weight. Talking with a family member, close friend, or counselor can help you see your problems in a new light. You might realize you are not alone or that your worries are normal.

On the flip side, spending time with supportive people can lift your mood. If you enjoy group activities, consider joining a hobby class or community event. The key is to connect with people who are understanding. This does not mean you should seek pity, but sometimes talking out a concern can calm your mind.

Learning to Say "No"

Many people feel stressed because they take on more tasks than they can manage. They say "yes" to every request, worried about being seen as unhelpful. However, saying "no" when you must can protect your mental health. You do not have to be rude. A kind but firm refusal might sound like, "I'm sorry, but I won't be able to take on another project right now."

If that feels uncomfortable, practice short lines you can use ahead of time. Remember that you have the right to decide how to use your time. Overloading yourself does not help anyone in the long run, because burnout can lead to even bigger problems down the road.

Quick Stress-Busters

1. **Short Breaks**: Step outside for a minute or look out a window. A change of scene can reset your mood.
2. **Movement**: Stretch your arms, roll your shoulders, or wiggle your fingers to reduce tension.
3. **Scent**: Certain smells, like lavender or citrus, can calm the mind. Consider a small scented item at your desk.
4. **Music**: A short playlist of calming tunes can bring your heart rate down.
5. **Humor**: Watching a funny clip or reading a joke can break the cycle of stress. Laughing is a strong stress reliever.

These do not solve major problems, but they can help you cope in the moment. They prevent stress from piling up minute by minute.

Avoiding Common Pitfalls

- **Ignoring Warning Signs**: If you notice you are breathing fast or getting headaches, do not ignore them. They could be telling you it is time to slow down.
- **Constant Multitasking**: Trying to do several tasks at once might feel productive, but often it just leads to errors and higher stress.

- **Thinking Stress Will Disappear on Its Own**: While some issues do resolve with time, most require some action or at least a plan. Waiting too long can make matters worse.
- **Relying on Harmful Coping**: Some people turn to alcohol or other substances to cope. This might bring short relief but creates bigger problems later, including increased anxiety when the effect wears off.

Problem-Solving Approach

Sometimes stress comes from a problem that needs a real solution, like a financial shortfall or a conflict with a neighbor. In these cases, a clear plan can help:

1. **Define the Issue**: Be specific. "I'm short on rent this month."
2. **List Possible Solutions**: Brainstorm everything, even if it seems silly.
3. **Weigh Pros and Cons**: Look at each option and see which is best or doable.
4. **Pick One and Act**: Move forward with that choice. If it does not work, you can pick another.
5. **Evaluate**: Ask yourself what worked, what did not, and what you can learn.

Having a plan can lower the sense of dread. Even if the problem is not solved instantly, knowing you have steps to follow can reduce stress.

Long-Term Changes

Short-term tricks are great for quick relief. However, if you notice a pattern of stress, you may want to make bigger changes:

- **Cut Back on Over-Commitments**: Check your calendar and see if you can remove activities that do not bring real value.
- **Rethink Life Choices**: In some cases, an unfulfilling job or toxic relationship can cause constant stress. It might be time to consider changes.
- **Pace Yourself**: Set realistic goals for personal projects. Avoid trying to do too much at once.

- **Seek Guidance**: If stress relates to finances, health, or family, talking to a professional (like a financial advisor or counselor) could help you find a structured path.

Linking Stress Management with Anxiety Relief

Managing stress is closely tied to lowering anxiety. When the body and mind get used to dealing with stress in healthier ways, anxiety has less room to grow. Methods like breathing exercises, breaks, and boundary-setting not only reduce stress but also stop anxious thoughts from building up.

Tracking Your Stress Levels

Some people use a simple scale from 1 to 10 to rate their stress each day. Over time, they see patterns: maybe stress is highest on Monday mornings or after a certain type of event. This knowledge can help you plan. If Monday is always tough, you might schedule a calming walk or a friendly catch-up that day. Or you might do some prep work on Sunday evening to reduce Monday panic.

Journaling can also help. Jot down what happened on stressful days, how you felt, and what you tried. This can teach you which methods work best. You can then use those methods again in the future.

Adapting to Change

Life changes, both big and small, can bring stress. Even happy events like graduating or getting married can create pressure. One way to deal with big changes is to plan in stages. For example, if you are moving, list tasks such as packing, changing your address, and setting up your new place. Tackle them step by step. This reduces the sense of being swamped.

Also, accept that change usually comes with uncertainty. You cannot control every detail, but you can prepare for what is likely. Focus on what you can handle, rather than worrying about what might happen. This approach can lower the tension that arises from the unknown.

When Professional Help Is Needed

If stress feels unmanageable or is leading to severe anxiety, it may be time to seek professional advice. Signs include:

- Daily tasks feel impossible.
- Sleep is constantly disturbed.
- Appetite changes are extreme.
- You feel hopeless or deeply unhappy.

A therapist, counselor, or doctor can help find ways to reduce stress or suggest treatments for chronic anxiety. This does not mean you are weak. It means you recognize you need more tools than you currently have. Many people find that counseling or short-term medication can help them through a tough period.

Putting It All Together

Stress management is about finding balance. Life will always have pressures, but you do not have to be at their mercy. By learning how stress works, looking for early warning signs, and using practical methods like breaks, good time management, and supportive relationships, you can keep stress at levels you can handle. This, in turn, keeps anxiety from spinning out of control.

In the chapters so far, we have discussed what anxiety is, what signs to look for, what might cause it, how thoughts shape it, how self-talk can improve it, and now how to handle stress. Each piece fits into the bigger picture of mental health. In the upcoming chapters, we will continue to build on this foundation by exploring other topics like diet, sleep, and healthy routines.

By using stress management, you create a calmer environment for your body and mind. This helps reduce the cycle of worry that leads to anxiety. Think of stress management as daily upkeep for your mental well-being. With a few simple habits and a willingness to make changes, you can face life's pressures without feeling trapped by them. By taking action now, you can protect your future health and happiness,

CHAPTER 7: DIET AND EXERCISE

Diet and exercise play a big role in how we feel, both mentally and physically. When we are anxious, it can affect our eating habits and our desire to move. At the same time, what we eat and how we move our bodies can change our mood and how stressed we feel. In this chapter, we will look at how certain foods, nutrients, and types of exercise can help reduce anxiety. We will also look at some lesser-known ideas that might give you new ways to manage your well-being.

How Food Affects Mood

The brain is sensitive to what we eat. It relies on nutrients to produce chemicals that affect our mood. If we eat mostly junk food, we might feel tired or on edge. If we include helpful foods, we may feel calmer and more alert. Here are some ways diet and mood are linked:

1. **Blood Sugar Levels**: When we eat foods high in sugar, our blood sugar spikes and then crashes. This can lead to feelings of nervousness, shaking, or clouded thinking. Steady blood sugar helps keep the mind stable, so choosing whole grains and protein instead of sugary snacks can help avoid big ups and downs.
2. **Vitamins and Minerals**: Certain vitamins, like B vitamins and vitamin D, are important for a healthy nervous system. Low levels of B vitamins can lead to issues like restlessness or trouble focusing. Low vitamin D can affect mood and raise the risk of feeling sad or worried. Minerals like magnesium also help with muscle and nerve function. Not having enough magnesium can make stress feel worse.
3. **Healthy Fats**: Foods with good fats, such as fatty fish, avocados, and nuts, help maintain brain health. These fats can help reduce inflammation in the body, which can be linked to a tense mood. They also help the brain form connections needed for clear thinking.
4. **Protein**: Protein sources like chicken, beans, eggs, or fish contain amino acids. Some amino acids help the body create important brain chemicals. If you do not get enough protein, your body may lack these building blocks, which can lead to feeling more unsettled.
5. **Water Intake**: Dehydration can make you feel tired or confused, which can then add to anxiety. Even slight dehydration might affect mood. Drinking enough water helps your body handle stress.

Balanced Eating Tips

A balanced meal includes protein, whole grains, fruits, or vegetables, and healthy fats. It is not about strict diets or refusing favorite treats forever. It is about finding a steady way to fuel the body and brain:

1. **Do Not Skip Meals**: Skipping meals can cause a drop in blood sugar, which might lead to feeling jittery or worried. Even a small snack with protein and complex carbs (like a handful of nuts and a piece of fruit) can help keep energy stable.
2. **Plan Healthy Snacks**: If you know you get hungry in the afternoon, plan a snack like yogurt with fruit, or hummus with vegetable sticks. This helps you avoid grabbing candy or chips at the last minute.
3. **Limit Caffeine**: Caffeine in coffee, tea, or energy drinks can make some people feel more on edge. You do not have to quit caffeine entirely if you enjoy it, but pay attention to how it affects you. Maybe limit caffeine intake to mornings, so it does not disturb your sleep or raise your heart rate later in the day.
4. **Reduce High-Sugar Foods**: A sweet treat now and then is fine, but eating too many sugary foods can lead to blood sugar swings. Over time, this can contribute to mood changes or anxious feelings.
5. **Mindful Eating**: Try to notice the flavors and textures of your food. Eat slowly if possible. This can help you feel more relaxed and also help you notice when you are full. It is a simple way to reduce stress at mealtime.

Specific Nutrients Linked to Calmness

1. **Magnesium**: Found in foods like spinach, nuts, seeds, and whole grains. Low magnesium levels have been linked to tense muscles and trouble sleeping. Having enough magnesium might help the body handle stress better.
2. **Omega-3 Fatty Acids**: Found in fish like salmon, sardines, or in flaxseeds and walnuts. These fats help brain function and may lower inflammation. Studies suggest they can help with mood stability.
3. **Probiotics**: Found in some yogurts, kefir, or fermented vegetables. These foods support healthy gut bacteria, which is linked to better mood. Some research shows that a balanced gut can help reduce anxious thoughts.

4. **Complex Carbohydrates**: Found in oats, brown rice, or beans. They break down slowly, helping maintain steady energy and mood throughout the day.

While no single food is a magic fix, eating a variety of nutrient-rich foods can create a supportive base for your mind and body.

Lesser-Known Ideas About Food and Anxiety

- **Food Sensitivities**: Some people notice they feel more anxious after eating certain foods. This can be linked to sensitivities or intolerances. It might be worth keeping a food diary to see if certain items trigger anxious feelings.
- **Nutrient Timing**: Some find it helpful to eat small, balanced meals or snacks every few hours instead of three big meals. Spacing out food intake can keep blood sugar steady and reduce dips in energy.
- **Herbal Teas**: Teas like chamomile or peppermint can help some people feel more at ease. While this is not a cure, it can be a soothing part of a bedtime routine or a break during the day.

Exercise and Anxiety

Exercise is one of the most effective ways to reduce anxiety. It works by lowering stress hormones and increasing feel-good chemicals in the brain. It also helps distract the mind from worries. Here are some ways exercise can help:

1. **Physical Release**: Tension can build up in the body when we are worried. Exercise helps burn off that tension through movement.
2. **Better Sleep**: People who exercise regularly often sleep better. Good rest can reduce overall anxious feelings.
3. **Boosts Confidence**: Seeing that you can get stronger or improve in an activity can remind you that you can handle other challenges as well.
4. **Social Benefits**: If you join a class or group, you can meet others with similar goals. Social support can help reduce worry and negative thoughts.

Types of Exercise to Consider

1. **Aerobic Exercise**: This includes jogging, brisk walking, or cycling. Aerobic activities increase your heart rate, which helps use up stress hormones and improve heart health.
2. **Strength Training**: Lifting weights or doing bodyweight exercises can build muscle and bone strength. It can also help the body use energy in a calm, steady way.
3. **Yoga-Inspired Stretching**: Gentle stretches and poses help relax tense muscles. Some sequences also teach slow breathing, which can calm the mind.
4. **Short Movement Breaks**: If you are busy, small bursts of movement (like a quick walk around the block or a few squats by your desk) can still bring relief.
5. **Dancing**: Moving to music can be fun and help you forget worries for a bit. It also gets the heart pumping.

Try different forms of exercise to find what you like. If you do not enjoy an activity, it might be harder to stick with it. It is okay to start small. Even 10 minutes a day can make a difference over time.

Building a Practical Exercise Routine

1. **Pick Realistic Goals**: If you are new to exercise, it might not be wise to aim for a long run right away. Start with a short walk or a simple home workout. Build up gradually.
2. **Schedule It**: Put exercise into your calendar like you would an important appointment. This helps make it a regular part of your day.
3. **Combine with Daily Tasks**: If you struggle to find time, try linking exercise to normal activities. For example, walk to the store instead of driving, or do light stretching while watching TV.
4. **Reward Yourself**: After you complete a workout, do something small you enjoy (like reading a chapter of a book or listening to a favorite song). This can motivate you to keep going.
5. **Track Progress**: Jot down how you feel after each session. Over time, you might see that your mood is better on days you move more.

Overcoming Exercise Barriers

- **Energy Levels**: Anxiety can be draining, so you might feel too tired to exercise. Start with a gentle routine, like a slow walk, to show yourself you can still move even when tired.
- **Negative Thoughts**: You might think, "I'm not good at this." Remind yourself that exercise is for your own health, not a contest. Focus on how it helps your body and mind feel better.
- **Physical Limitations**: If you have joint pain or another health problem, look for low-impact choices such as swimming or seated exercises. Talk to a doctor if you are unsure which activities are safe.
- **Time**: Many people say they do not have time to work out. But even small breaks for stretching or walking can help. Try to fit in quick movements here or there.

Balancing Diet and Exercise

Both diet and exercise work best if you see them as connected. When you eat well, you have more energy to exercise. When you move regularly, you might be more aware of what foods help you feel better:

- **Fuel Your Workout**: Have a small snack with carbs and protein (like a banana with peanut butter) before exercise if you are hungry. This can help you avoid feeling weak or dizzy.
- **Replenish After**: A light meal with protein and some complex carbs after exercise can help muscles recover.
- **Stay Hydrated**: Drink water before, during, and after exercise. Sweating can make you lose fluids, and staying hydrated aids clear thinking.

Eating Disorders and Excessive Exercise

Sometimes, in a desire to lower anxiety, people might go too far with diet or exercise. They might restrict food too much or exercise to the point of exhaustion. These behaviors can create more stress and can harm the body and mind:

- **Warning Signs**: Rapid weight loss, feeling guilty after eating, or feeling you must work out to "earn" food can be signs of an unhealthy approach.
- **Getting Help**: If you see these signs in yourself or someone else, it might be time to talk to a mental health professional. You deserve a balanced relationship with food and exercise.
- **Healthy Balance**: A healthy diet does not mean never eating treats. It means getting enough nutrients overall. A healthy exercise routine does not mean pushing until collapse, but rather finding a level that feels good and supports health.

Extra Factors

1. **Sunlight**: Getting outside can help the body produce vitamin D and can also lift mood. If you combine exercise with time in nature, you might get double benefits.
2. **Social Eating**: Sharing meals with friends or family can lower tension. It can also encourage slower eating. If you often eat alone or in a hurry, you might try sitting with someone you trust for a calm meal now and then.
3. **Preparation**: Planning meals ahead or doing light cooking in batches can reduce stress if you have busy days. It makes it easier to stick to balanced eating.
4. **Listen to Your Body**: If you feel hungry, consider what kind of hunger it is. Are you hungry for something warm and filling, or are you just bored? Learning these signals can prevent eating for the wrong reasons. The same goes for exercise—if you feel pain or strong fatigue, it might be time to rest or do a gentler form of movement.

Case Examples (Brief and Simple)

1. **Case of Carla**: Carla found that when she ate sugary snacks in the afternoon, she had a burst of energy but then felt shaky and worried an hour later. She began replacing these snacks with nuts and a piece of fruit. Over a few weeks, her afternoon worries became less strong. She also felt steadier energy at work.
2. **Case of Mike**: Mike felt he had no time to work out. He decided to walk during his lunch break instead of sitting in the break room. He started

with just 10 minutes each day. After a month, he realized his mood was better, and he looked forward to these walks. He then increased to 15 minutes and felt even calmer in the afternoons.

These small changes show that diet and exercise do not have to be huge or extreme. Minor adjustments can have noticeable benefits over time.

Practical Tips for Getting Started

- **Meal Planner**: Write down simple meal ideas for the week. Aim for a vegetable or fruit at each meal.
- **Snack Prep**: Keep easy, healthy snacks on hand. Wash and chop some vegetables or keep small bags of nuts ready.
- **Movement Choice**: Pick one short physical activity you like (like dancing in your living room or taking a slow jog). Put it on your schedule at least three times this week.
- **Track Changes**: Use a journal to note how you feel before and after eating better or doing a workout. Look for patterns in stress or anxiety levels.
- **Buddy Up**: If you have a friend who also wants to reduce stress, plan a walk or a simple cooking session together. Sharing the experience can keep you both motivated.

The Mind-Body Link

Healthy eating and regular exercise can send positive signals to the brain. Over time, these signals can reduce anxiety levels. While they may not eliminate anxiety completely, they build a more stable base for your overall well-being. A balanced diet supports the body's chemistry, and exercise lets out the tension that gathers in muscles during stressful times.

Warnings and Sensible Limits

- **Overexertion**: If you start a new workout plan, do not jump into very intense routines right away. Overdoing it can lead to injury and frustration.

- **Medical Conditions**: If you have ongoing health issues, talk to a health professional about which foods or workouts are best for you.
- **No Quick Fixes**: Neither diet nor exercise alone is a cure for anxiety. They are part of a bigger strategy that includes better thinking patterns, handling stress well, and other parts of self-care.
- **Progress, Not Perfection**: You might have days when you eat something that upsets your stomach or skip a workout. That does not ruin your overall effort. Aim for steady improvement rather than 100% perfect habits.

Combining Diet and Exercise with Other Steps

Chapters before this one covered how to handle stress, how to use good self-talk, and how to replace negative thinking. Diet and exercise link closely with all of these. For example, if you are managing stress better, you may feel more energy to cook healthier meals. If your self-talk is improving, you might be less likely to scold yourself for missing a workout and more likely to just get back on track the next day.

Many find that small improvements in one area create a positive chain reaction in other areas. That is the power of a well-rounded plan for mental health.

Looking Ahead

As you keep learning about yourself, pay attention to which foods make you feel calmer or more energetic. Note which activities help your mood and which ones feel too hard or stressful. Over time, you can shape a plan that fits well into your life. This plan might look different from someone else's plan, and that is okay. The main point is to support your mind and body in a way that feels right for you.

With diet and exercise in place, you will be better prepared to face challenges without feeling helpless. Good nutrition and regular movement can set the stage for a calmer mind. This does not mean you will never feel anxious. But it can mean you experience less severe worry, and you can recover faster when anxious feelings appear.

CHAPTER 8: SLEEP AND RELAXATION

Sleep and relaxation are often overlooked when people talk about managing worry. Yet they are critical for mental health. Lack of good rest can increase anxious thoughts, and proper relaxation can settle a tense mind and body. This chapter will explore the effects of sleep on stress, how relaxation can help, and lesser-known methods to improve both. You will also learn practical ways to wind down after a busy day and reduce anxious thoughts at bedtime.

Why Sleep Matters for Anxiety

1. **Brain Recovery**: When we sleep, the brain sorts out memories and resets certain chemical levels. If this process is cut short, the brain can remain in a stressed state.
2. **Hormone Regulation**: Sleep helps regulate hormones like cortisol, which is involved in stress. Without enough rest, cortisol levels can stay too high, adding to feelings of worry.
3. **Mental Energy**: A tired mind is less able to handle daily challenges. Small problems seem huge when we are exhausted. Over time, this can lead to constant strain.
4. **Emotional Balance**: During certain sleep phases, the brain processes emotions. Missing these phases can make it harder to handle stress or frustration.

Signs of Poor Sleep

- **Difficulty Falling Asleep**: Tossing and turning for more than 30 minutes or an hour most nights.
- **Frequent Waking**: Waking up many times during the night and finding it hard to go back to sleep.
- **Feeling Tired on Waking**: You slept long enough, but still feel exhausted in the morning.
- **Mood Swings**: Poor sleep can cause irritability, sadness, or anxious moods.
- **Increased Use of Stimulants**: Needing a lot of caffeine or sugar during the day to keep going.

If you notice these signs regularly, it might be time to pay closer attention to sleep habits. Improving them can significantly lower daily worry.

Common Sleep Disturbances Tied to Anxiety

1. **Racing Thoughts**: You lie down and suddenly your mind is busy, thinking of what happened today or what might happen tomorrow.
2. **Night Worries**: Small concerns can feel bigger in the quiet of night. The mind may replay past events or imagine worst-case scenarios.
3. **Physical Tension**: Tight muscles, a pounding heart, or shallow breathing can keep you from falling asleep.
4. **Waking Up Early**: Anxiety can sometimes cause people to wake up before the alarm, feeling uneasy and unable to return to sleep.

Improving Sleep Hygiene

Sleep hygiene refers to habits that help you get better rest. Here are key points:

1. **Consistent Bedtime**: Go to bed and wake up at the same time each day, even on weekends if possible. This sets your internal clock.
2. **Limit Screen Time Before Bed**: The light from phones and TVs can trick your body into staying awake. Try to stop using screens an hour before sleep.
3. **Bedroom Environment**: Keep the room cool, dark, and quiet. If there is noise from outside, consider earplugs or a white noise machine.
4. **Avoid Heavy Meals Before Sleep**: If you eat a large or spicy meal late at night, it can cause discomfort or heartburn. A small, light snack is usually okay.
5. **Reduce Caffeine**: Caffeine can stay in your system for hours. Try not to drink coffee or strong tea later in the day.
6. **Relaxing Routine**: Do a calm activity before bed, such as reading (a light or calm book), gentle stretching, or listening to soft music. This signals your brain that it is time to slow down.

Handling Nighttime Anxiety

- **Write It Down**: Keep a small notepad by your bed. If a worry pops up, jot it down. This can free your mind from holding onto it.
- **Picture a Calm Scene**: Imagine a place that feels safe, noticing details like colors or sounds. This can help shift focus away from worries.
- **Breathing Exercise**: Try a short breathing drill where you inhale for a count of four, hold for one or two seconds, then exhale for four. Focus on the rhythm rather than anxious thoughts.
- **Progressive Relaxation**: Tense and relax muscles starting from your toes up to your head. This method helps the body release stored tension.

If you cannot sleep after 20 or 30 minutes, get out of bed and do a calm activity in low light. Return to bed when you feel sleepy. This stops you from associating the bed with frustration and restlessness.

Relaxation Practices for Any Time

Relaxation does not only happen at night. You can practice calming methods during the day to lower overall tension:

1. **Breath Awareness**: Take a few minutes to notice your breathing. If it is quick or shallow, guide it to be slower and deeper.
2. **Body Scan**: Close your eyes and mentally check each part of your body from head to toe. Notice areas of tightness and let them relax.
3. **Gentle Stretching**: This can be done at work, school, or at home. Roll your shoulders, stretch your neck, or reach your arms overhead.
4. **Music or Nature Sounds**: Soft background sounds can help slow an overactive mind. Choose tunes that are not distracting.
5. **Short Breaks**: Take small 5-minute rests in between tasks. Stand up, move around, and let your mind recharge.

These practices help break the cycle of stress buildup. The calmer your day is, the easier it can be to fall asleep at night.

Less-Known Methods for Better Rest

1. **Foot Soak or Warm Shower**: Raising your body temperature slightly and then letting it cool can trigger a sleepy feeling. A warm foot soak or short shower might help you relax.
2. **Aromatherapy**: Scents like lavender or chamomile can help some people feel calm. You could use a small diffuser or a scented pillow.
3. **Weighted Blanket**: Some people find that a slightly heavier blanket helps them feel secure, reducing tossing and turning.
4. **Cool Bedroom Temperature**: The body sleeps best in a slightly cool environment. Experiment with thermostat settings or a fan.

Relaxation and the Mind

Anxiety often comes from a fast-moving mind. Relaxation is like training the mind to slow down. Think of it as teaching yourself to flip a switch from "go" to "rest." This can be tricky at first because many of us stay in "go" mode all day. But with practice, you can learn to shift gears:

- **Practice at Calm Times**: Do not wait until you are very anxious to practice. Try a relaxation drill when you already feel okay, so you build skill.
- **Stay Consistent**: Even if you do not feel instantly relaxed, keep at it. The mind needs time to form new habits.
- **Accept Ups and Downs**: Some days, a relaxation method might work great. Other days, it might not. This is normal. Just keep using healthy steps.

Connecting Relaxation with Other Anxiety Methods

If you have read earlier chapters, you know about self-talk and stress management. Relaxation fits neatly with them:

- **Self-Talk**: As you relax, you can remind yourself with calm words: "I'm safe right now. I can let my muscles rest."

- **Stress Management**: Handling stress during the day means you have less stress to calm at night. If you set boundaries or manage time well, your mind is less overloaded at bedtime.
- **Physical Exercise**: Exercise can help you feel pleasantly tired at night, making relaxation easier. Just try to avoid vigorous exercise right before bedtime, as it may keep you awake.

Creating a Bedtime Routine

A bedtime routine signals the body that it is time to sleep. It can be brief or longer, depending on your schedule. For example:

1. **Lower the Lights**: Bright lights can make the mind think it is still daytime. Dim lamps help the brain wind down.
2. **Put Devices Away**: Stop checking email or messages. This lowers mental stimulation.
3. **Gentle Activity**: You might do a bit of gentle stretching or read a calm book.
4. **Quiet Reflection**: Take a moment to note something from the day that you are thankful for. This can shift the mind away from worries.
5. **Lights Out**: Once you feel relaxed, turn off the light. Try a breathing exercise if thoughts keep coming.

Dealing with Insomnia

If you have insomnia that lasts for weeks or more, it might be time to seek professional help. Possible causes can include health conditions, medication side effects, or severe anxiety disorders. A doctor or counselor can look at your sleep habits and suggest treatments like cognitive behavioral therapy for insomnia (CBT-I). This method helps change thoughts and behaviors around sleep.

Relaxation for Daytime Anxiety

You do not have to wait until evening to relax. Many people feel anxious in the middle of the day. Quick exercises can help:

- **Coloring or Simple Drawing**: If you enjoy art, a short coloring break can calm the mind.
- **Hand Massage**: Gently rubbing your hands with lotion or oil can relax tense muscles.
- **Sensory Techniques**: Focus on one sense at a time. Look for three things you see, two things you touch, and one thing you hear. This can ground you in the present moment.

Combining Relaxation with Professional Guidance

For serious or long-standing anxiety, a mental health professional can guide you to relax effectively. They might teach special forms of therapy that include relaxation. This can be helpful if you find it hard to calm down by yourself or if anxiety is linked to deeper issues. Sometimes a short course of medication might help you regain a normal sleep pattern, though that decision should be made with a doctor.

Tech Tools for Better Sleep and Relaxation

While it is wise to limit screen time near bedtime, there are still tools that can help you in other parts of the day:

1. **Meditation Apps**: Some apps offer guided breathing or calming stories. Just be sure to turn them off well before lights out.
2. **Sleep Trackers**: Wearable devices can log how much you toss and turn, giving you data to see if your habits are helping or hurting.
3. **Calm Music Playlists**: Platforms with playlists designed to help with rest can be a good aid. Remember to keep the volume low.
4. **White Noise Machines**: These devices produce a steady, neutral sound that can mask other noises.

Avoiding Common Sleep Mistakes

- **Oversleeping on Weekends**: Sleeping far beyond your normal time can disrupt your sleep cycle. If you need extra rest, try an afternoon nap instead of sleeping until noon.

- **Using Bed for Non-Sleep Activities**: Working, studying, or watching intense shows in bed trains your mind to be active there. Keep the bed for rest and calm moments if you can.
- **Late Heavy Workouts**: Exercising late can raise the body's temperature and alertness, making it tough to wind down. If you must exercise late, do a gentle form like light stretches or a slow walk.
- **Clock-Watching**: Checking the time repeatedly can add to worry. Turn the clock away so you are not tempted to look at it when you cannot sleep.

A Look at Naps

Naps can help if you did not sleep well at night or if you have a midday energy drop. But long naps, especially late in the day, might ruin night sleep. A short nap of about 20-30 minutes earlier in the afternoon can be refreshing. If you nap too close to bedtime, it might be harder to fall asleep at night.

Putting Relaxation into Daily Life

Relaxation should not be a chore. Think of it as a friendly pause for your mind and body. You could do a small breathing practice before starting your car or while waiting in a line. You might set a gentle reminder on your phone to pause for a quick body scan. Over time, these small breaks create a habit of calm. They train the mind to return to a steady state instead of staying in stress mode.

Progress and Patience

Improving sleep and relaxation is like training a muscle. It may take a few weeks or even months to see strong results. You might still have nights when you struggle to rest. That is okay. The goal is to reduce these rough nights and give your body more opportunities to reset. Keep track of what helps and what does not. Tweak your approach as you learn more about your own patterns.

Summary of Key Points

- **Sleep**: Aim for consistency, a calm environment, and a relaxing routine.
- **Relaxation**: Practice calming techniques during the day so it is easier at night.
- **Nighttime Anxiety**: Write worries down, try gentle breathing, or do short relaxation drills.
- **Environment**: A cool, dark, and quiet bedroom supports deeper rest.
- **Daily Stress**: Lower overall stress through quick breaks and good time management. This helps prevent bedtime anxiety.
- **Seek Help if Needed**: If insomnia persists, talk to a professional.

Looking Forward

Sleep and relaxation are powerful parts of handling anxiety. They allow the body and mind to recover so we can face each day with more peace. When combined with other methods like balanced eating, exercise, and good self-talk, they form a strong shield against overwhelming worry.

In the next chapter, we will explore healthy routines that bring everything together—stress management, diet, exercise, and rest. By building daily habits that work well for you, you can give yourself the best chance of feeling calm and in control. Good sleep and relaxation are not luxuries; they are the foundation that supports a calmer mind.

A well-rested body and mind can handle more challenges, whether they come from work, family, or life changes. By giving attention to sleep and relaxation, you show care for your overall health. It may feel odd to spend time on something that seems passive, but rest is an active part of self-care. As you refine your bedtime routine and relax during the day, you may notice that anxious thoughts carry less weight. You can then use your energy for the things that matter to you, rather than being drained by worry.

CHAPTER 9: HEALTHY ROUTINES

Having a healthy routine can shape how you feel day after day. A healthy routine does not mean a boring life or a rigid schedule with no fun. It means setting up habits that support a calmer mind and a stronger body. For people dealing with anxiety, such routines can keep stress from climbing too high. In this chapter, we will look at several angles of building daily structure, from morning to evening. We will include practical ideas that are not commonly discussed, giving you fresh ways to care for your well-being.

Why Routines Help with Anxiety

Routines give a sense of predictability. When life feels chaotic, simple habits—like regular bedtimes, set mealtimes, or planned breaks—can give the mind a safe anchor. Rather than feeling lost, you know at least part of your day follows a steady pattern. This can reduce mental strain. Also, routines can prevent you from forgetting key tasks, which might otherwise cause last-minute stress.

Moreover, routines help preserve mental energy. If every part of your day is random, you end up making many small decisions ("Should I eat now or later?" "Should I exercise in the morning or at night?"). Decision-making can be tiring when done all the time. A basic structure removes some of that burden, letting you save energy for bigger challenges.

Morning Habits for a Calm Start

1. **Wake-Up Time**
   A consistent wake-up time trains your internal clock. If you wake up at very different times each day, your body might struggle to know when to release energy hormones. Setting a morning alarm at roughly the same time helps regulate mood and energy.
2. **Sunlight**
   Getting daylight early in the morning sends signals to the brain that it is time to be alert. If possible, open a window or step outside for a few

minutes. This helps stabilize your internal clock and can help you feel more awake without needing too much caffeine.

3. **Gentle Movement**
   Some people enjoy a short stretch routine or a slow walk. It does not have to be a full workout—just enough to warm your muscles and gently boost blood flow. This can help clear morning grogginess and prepare you for the day.
4. **Mindful Moment**
   Before checking messages or social media, take a minute to notice your thoughts. Are you feeling worried about something today? Maybe you can list one thing you look forward to. This small pause can help guide your day in a more balanced direction.
5. **Simple Breakfast**
   If your body feels shaky in the morning, a little protein and some healthy carbohydrates can make a big difference. Try a banana with peanut butter, or some eggs with whole-grain toast. This helps prevent blood sugar dips that might trigger anxious feelings later.

Planning Your Day

After your morning routine, it can help to outline the day's tasks. A to-do list, written or in a simple app, can prevent random thoughts about "What am I forgetting?" This is especially useful for those prone to worry. Here are some points to keep in mind:

- **Set Realistic Tasks**: Avoid overstuffing the list. A long, impossible list can create more tension.
- **Prioritize**: Put the most important or urgent tasks at the top. That way, if you run out of time, at least the main tasks are done.
- **Flexible Blocks**: Leave some open time for breaks or unplanned events. This prevents panic if something unexpected appears.
- **Reward System**: If you finish a tough task, give yourself a small reward, like reading a few pages of a book, enjoying a piece of fruit you like, or chatting with a friend for a minute.

This structure helps you feel in control of your day, which can lead to lower anxiety overall.

Work and Study Routines

Many people feel anxiety in work or school settings. A stable work or study routine can reduce tension:

1. **Focused Sessions**
   Instead of working non-stop, try time blocks. Work for 25-30 minutes on a task, then take a 5-minute break to stand up or stretch. This approach can keep the mind fresh. It also reduces the overwhelming feeling of one long work session.
2. **Clear Boundaries**
   If possible, separate your work area from your relaxation area. Even if you only have one room, designate a corner or desk where you do your tasks. This trains your brain to work there and relax elsewhere.
3. **Regular Check-Ins**
   If you have a long project, break it into stages. Check your progress at set intervals—maybe at midday and near the end of the day. This prevents tasks from piling up and turning into a huge problem later.
4. **Healthy Work Snacks**
   Long study or work sessions can cause you to grab something sugary out of habit. Instead, keep better options at hand, like nuts, yogurt, or fruit. This keeps you fueled without the crash that often follows a sugar high.
5. **Set an End Time**
   Anxiety can rise if work or study seems never-ending. If possible, pick a cut-off time in the evening. After that, allow yourself to step away. Overworking can harm mental health. Stopping at a set time can reduce guilt about taking breaks.

Afternoon Adjustments

The afternoon slump is common. Energy can dip, making anxiety more noticeable. Here are ways to handle that:

1. **Brief Movement Break**
   Even a 10-minute walk outside or around the office can raise your energy. It also gives your mind a chance to recharge. If you can't go outside, some light stretching by your desk or in a hallway can still help.

2. **Check Hydration**
   By midday, many forget to drink water. Slight dehydration can cause tiredness and restlessness. A glass of water can be a quick fix.
3. **Light Snack**
   If there are still hours until dinner, a balanced snack can keep blood sugar stable. Look for something with protein and complex carbs, such as a whole-grain cracker with cheese or hummus with veggies.
4. **Short Calm Pause**
   If you feel worries building up, pause and close your eyes for a few deep breaths. Notice how your shoulders feel. Are they tight? Relax them. This quick reset can prevent anxiety from escalating.

Evening Habits for Wind-Down

1. **Transition from Work**
   If you work from home, try to put away laptops or files at a set time. Change into comfortable clothing. This signals your mind that the workday is over. If you commute, use the travel time to listen to relaxing music or a soothing podcast.
2. **Supper Choices**
   A healthy evening meal should not be too heavy. Large, greasy meals or very spicy food right before bedtime can disrupt sleep. Consider a balanced meal with vegetables, protein, and perhaps a bit of healthy fat, like avocado or olive oil.
3. **Lower Lights**
   Dim the lights in your home as it gets later. Bright lights can trick the brain into thinking it is still daytime. This small change in lighting can support natural sleep cues.
4. **Unplug Early**
   If possible, stop checking work emails or social media an hour before bedtime. This can help reduce the mental chatter that often leads to late-night tossing and turning.
5. **Calming Activities**
   Consider reading a lighthearted book, listening to gentle music, or enjoying a warm drink (non-caffeinated). Some find a short warm bath helps them relax. It is a matter of personal preference.

Anchors on Tough Days

Sometimes, despite good routines, anxiety can spike. Maybe you got unexpected news or you are facing a challenging deadline. Having "anchor tasks" can be a safety net on those days:

- **Anchor 1**: A quick breathing exercise that steadies the heart rate. Doing it in the bathroom or a private corner can help you return to a calm baseline.
- **Anchor 2**: A short text or call to someone supportive. Just hearing a calm voice can reduce panic.
- **Anchor 3**: A moment of stillness. Step outside, close your eyes, and listen to your surroundings. Even 60 seconds can be enough to reduce a surge of worry.

These anchors do not solve all problems, but they can stop anxiety from getting out of control and messing up the entire day.

Weekly Structure

A healthy routine is not just about daily habits, but also about weekly planning. Here are ideas for weekly structure:

1. **Meal Planning**
   Spending a bit of time each weekend planning meals can lower stress on busy weekdays. You do not need to cook everything in advance, but having ingredients and ideas ready prevents last-minute panic.
2. **Chore Distribution**
   Instead of letting chores pile up, try assigning certain tasks to certain days. For example, laundry on Wednesday, cleaning the kitchen on Saturday. Spreading out tasks can prevent weekend overload.
3. **Hobby or Fun Activity**
   Set at least one day or evening for something you enjoy, such as painting, reading, or playing a sport. Protect that time as much as possible. Knowing you have a fun activity planned can ease weekday stress.
4. **Review and Reset**
   At the end of the week, review what went well and what caused stress. Make small changes for the next week. This consistent reflection can help you adjust your routines so they stay useful.

Social Routines

Loneliness can increase anxiety. Building social routines can help:

1. **Regular Catch-Ups**
   Plan a quick phone call or coffee with a friend once a week or so. A brief chat can keep connections strong.
2. **Group Activities**
   Joining a regular group activity, like a club or volunteer team, gives you something to look forward to. It also helps form new friendships, which can reduce feelings of isolation.
3. **Family Time**
   If you live with family, set a shared meal where everyone sits together without devices. It might be once a week if daily is not possible. This can strengthen bonds and reduce tension that builds when people do not communicate.

Digital Device Habits

Phones and computers can be a source of stress. Creating a routine for device use can protect mental health:

1. **Notification Management**
   Turn off non-essential notifications. Constant pings can feed anxiety. Maybe set specific times to check email or social media instead of checking them all day.
2. **Screen-Free Zones**
   If possible, pick a spot in your home, such as the dining table or bedroom, where you do not use devices. This helps you separate online time from offline rest.
3. **Night Mode**
   Many devices have a "night mode" that changes screen colors to reduce harsh light in the evening. This can help your eyes and brain wind down. Still, it is best to limit screen time close to bedtime.

Rethinking Weekends

Weekends often bring a different schedule. Some people fill them with errands or social events. Others stay in bed all day. A middle path can be more helpful:

- **Keep Wake-Up Time Close**
  Sleeping a bit more on weekends can feel nice, but going from 6 a.m. on weekdays to noon on weekends can confuse your internal clock. Aim to keep your wake-up time within an hour or so of your weekday schedule.
- **Plan One Fun Event**
  Give yourself something enjoyable. It might be a visit to a park or cooking a new recipe. This can refresh your mind for the week ahead.
- **Set Chores**
  If you use weekends for chores, plan them in smaller chunks instead of one huge block. This allows for rest or mini-breaks.
- **Unplug Time**
  If you can, put away work emails. Let your mind have a real break so you do not start Monday already exhausted.

Handling Interruptions

Life can disrupt the best routines. Maybe you get sick or a friend calls with an emergency. Try these steps when routines get shaken:

1. **Address the Urgent Issue First**
   If it is a true emergency, do what is needed. Do not feel guilty about ignoring your usual plan on these days.
2. **Return to Basics**
   Once things calm down, return to your basic routine as soon as possible. For example, keep your regular bedtime even if you skipped some other habits.
3. **Gentle Self-Talk**
   Remind yourself that life changes happen. Missing a planned workout or meal does not ruin everything. Aim for consistency over time, not day-by-day perfection.
4. **Communicate**
   If someone else's emergency is pulling on your schedule, let them know your limits. While you want to help, you also need to protect your mental well-being.

Lesser-Known Tips for Routine Building

1. **Habit Stacking**
   Link a new habit to something you already do. For instance, if you want to start reading a self-help passage daily, place the book on top of your phone at night. In the morning, when you reach for the phone, you see the book and remember to read.
2. **Create "If-Then" Plans**
   Plan for possible disruptions. "If I cannot get home in time to cook dinner, I will have a simple sandwich and a vegetable side instead of ordering fast food." This prevents panic decisions.
3. **Use Visual Reminders**
   Sticky notes on the fridge or a simple chart on your wall can keep your new habits in sight. This helps you stay focused on what you decided to do.
4. **Track It**
   Some people find it helpful to use a daily habit tracker (on paper or an app). Each day you complete a habit, you mark it. This simple act can motivate you to keep going.

Balancing Flexibility and Routine

A routine should not become a source of stress by being too rigid. Balance is key:

- **Allow Some Choices**
  If every moment is scheduled, you might feel trapped. Instead, set broad blocks of time for tasks. For example, "Sometime between 8 and 9 a.m., I'll do my small stretching." That way, you still have freedom.
- **Leave Room for Fun**
  Make sure there is time for hobbies, relaxation, or hanging out with friends. If every second is work or chores, you could feel burnt out.
- **Review Often**
  Every couple of weeks, assess if your routine is still working. If you find certain habits are not helpful, adjust them. The goal is to support your mental health, not to follow a set plan just because you wrote it.

Benefits of a Well-Tuned Routine

1. **Stability**
   Knowing what to expect can reduce the feeling of being overwhelmed. Small changes are easier to handle when you have a solid foundation.
2. **Better Sleep**
   Consistent routines often lead to better bedtime habits. This translates into deeper rest and less morning anxiety.
3. **Improved Focus**
   When your day is well-organized, you can devote full attention to tasks. This helps you complete them faster, lowering the chance of last-minute rush.
4. **Reduced Decision Fatigue**
   With some decisions made in advance (like meal plans or workout slots), you do not waste mental energy on small questions repeatedly.
5. **Healthier Lifestyle**
   Over time, good routines around diet, movement, and rest can boost overall health. A healthy body can help the mind stay more balanced.

Checking In on Your Progress

Routines need monitoring to see if they are truly helping. Every week or two, you might ask:

- "Did I feel more calm this week than last?"
- "Which part of the routine did I skip or forget?"
- "Did that skipping affect my anxiety?"
- "Are there any new stressors that need me to adjust the routine?"

Be honest about what works or what feels forced. The aim is steady improvement, not perfection.

Tips for Overcoming Obstacles

- **Start Small**: If you do not have a routine at all, begin with one or two simple changes, like a set bedtime or a 15-minute walk in the morning.

- **Buddy System**: If you have a friend or family member who also wants a routine, share your goals with each other. You can check in once a week for support.
- **Self-Compassion**: If you miss a habit or get off track, do not beat yourself up. Everyone stumbles. Just refocus the next day.

Golden Gems for Routines

Here are some less usual but helpful ideas:

1. **Theme Days**
   Assign a theme to certain days. For instance, Monday might be "organize day," when you tidy or plan. Tuesday could be "learning day," when you watch an educational video or read new material. This can add variety and a sense of fun structure to your week.
2. **Micro-Chores**
   Instead of a big cleaning day, tackle a "micro-chore" each day that takes just five minutes, like wiping a shelf or sorting a small stack of papers. Over time, these add up, lowering your weekend chore load and daily mess stress.
3. **Desk Stretch Cards**
   Create or print small cards with simple stretches you can do at your desk. Every hour or two, pick a card and do that stretch. This keeps your body from tightening up during long work sessions.
4. **Wind-Down Alarm**
   We use alarms to wake up, but an alarm can also remind you when it is time to slow down at night. Set it 30 minutes before bedtime. Once it rings, wrap up what you are doing and start your bedtime routine.

Putting It All Together

Building a healthy routine is like putting together pieces of a puzzle. Each piece—morning habits, work methods, evening wind-down—contributes to an overall picture of stability. Once your puzzle is mostly complete, anxiety finds fewer cracks to slip through. You might still have stressful days, but your routine gives you a framework to handle them. The predictability can calm your mind, and the healthy habits can keep your body in good shape.

CHAPTER 10: PANIC AND FEAR

Panic and fear can catch people by surprise. One moment, things seem fine; the next, the heart is pounding, the body is shaky, and the mind is gripped by terror. Some people experience panic attacks, which can be brief but intense episodes of feeling overwhelmed by dread. Others face specific fears, like fear of heights, fear of social situations, or fear of losing control. In this chapter, we will look at what panic and fear really are, why they appear, and how to respond when they show up. We will also offer some practical ideas that might not be common, giving you new ways to handle these strong emotions.

What Is Panic?

Panic is a sudden spike in anxiety that can bring strong physical signs such as:

- Racing heartbeat
- Sweating
- Shortness of breath
- Chest tightness or pain
- Dizziness
- Trembling
- An intense sense that something horrible is about to happen

A panic attack usually lasts a few minutes to half an hour, though it can feel much longer. The person might think they are having a heart attack or that they are losing their mind. Often, after the first panic attack, a new fear forms: the fear of having another attack. This can lead to avoidance of places or situations where panic once appeared.

What Is Fear?

Fear is a response to something the mind labels as threatening. Unlike panic, which can strike suddenly, fear might build over time. It could be a fear of dogs, public speaking, closed spaces, or flying. Fear can also be less specific, like a fear of embarrassment in social settings or a fear of failing at a task.

While fear itself is not bad—often it keeps us safe from real danger—sometimes it arises even when the danger is not truly severe or is only a small possibility. That is where fear becomes a problem. If fear stops you from normal activities, it can damage quality of life.

Why Do Panic and Fear Happen?

1. **Body's Alarm System**
   Humans evolved to respond quickly to threats. Adrenaline and other hormones flood the body, preparing it to fight or run. This is useful if a wild animal is chasing you, but less useful if you are simply waiting for a train or about to give a short talk at work.
2. **Past Experiences**
   A previous frightening event can teach the mind to expect panic in similar situations. This can happen with car accidents, medical emergencies, or even humiliating social moments.
3. **Genetic Tendency**
   Some people have a body that is more sensitive to signals of threat. They might get startled more easily or take longer to calm down.
4. **Learned Responses**
   If you saw a parent or sibling react with great fear to certain things, you might learn to do the same. Fear can spread within families or social circles.

The Cycle of Panic

Panic can form a loop:

1. You notice a physical sign (like a faster heartbeat).
2. You think, "I'm in danger," even if there is no real threat.
3. Your body releases more stress hormones, increasing heart rate and tension.
4. You become more convinced something terrible is happening.
5. Panic grows until it peaks.

The cycle feeds on itself. The key is often to break it early by recognizing that the physical signs do not always mean real danger.

Handling a Panic Attack in the Moment

1. **Grounding Technique**
   Name five things you can see, four things you can touch, three things you can hear, two you can smell, and one you can taste or sense. This can shift your focus away from internal fear to the outside world.
2. **Belly Breathing**
   Slow your breathing by inhaling gently through your nose, letting your stomach expand, then exhaling slowly through your mouth. Count the seconds to make it regular. This can help reset the body's alarm.
3. **Reassuring Self-Talk**
   Remind yourself, "I've been through this before, and it passed," or "My body is reacting to stress, but I am not in real danger." Repeating calm words can lower panic's intensity.
4. **Focus on an Object**
   Find something in the room or area—maybe a picture or a small item in your pocket—and study it closely. This gives your brain a concrete, safe task, weakening the panic spiral.
5. **Seek a Supportive Person**
   If possible, talk to a friend or family member. Hearing a calm voice can help. Even if you just tell them you feel a bit panicky, that sharing can lower the sense of isolation.

Long-Term Strategies for Panic

1. **Therapy**
   Certain types of counseling, like cognitive-behavioral therapy (CBT), can teach you to recognize and change thought patterns that lead to panic. Therapists might also use exposure methods where you gradually face the triggers in a safe way.
2. **Relaxation Training**
   Regular practice of breathing exercises or muscle relaxation can make you more skilled at calming down when panic starts.
3. **Physical Health**
   Keeping up with a balanced diet, exercise, and enough sleep helps the body manage stress better. A tense, tired body is more prone to panic.
4. **Medication**
   In some cases, a doctor may prescribe short-term or long-term

medication to lower the intensity of panic. This choice depends on personal and medical factors. Medication does not solve everything, but it can give you room to work on coping skills.
5. **Support Groups**
Talking to others who have had panic attacks can reduce the feeling that you are alone. Groups (online or in person) can offer encouragement and new tips.

Specific Fears (Phobias)

Phobias are intense fears of specific objects or situations, such as spiders, flying, or heights. These can lead to avoidance that disrupts life. Methods to handle phobias include:

1. **Gradual Exposure**
Under guidance or with a plan, you slowly face the feared object or situation. For example, someone afraid of dogs might start by looking at pictures of dogs, then watching them from afar, then petting a calm dog. Over time, the fear often shrinks.
2. **Visualization**
Imagining yourself handling the feared situation calmly. This trains the mind to link the situation with a calmer response.
3. **Breathing and Relaxation**
Using calming techniques right before and during exposure to keep the body from going into full panic. With practice, you learn you can face the fear without catastrophe happening.
4. **Getting Facts**
Sometimes understanding more about what you fear reduces the unknown. For instance, learning about how airplanes are maintained might help someone with flight anxiety see that the real risk is lower than they imagined.

Social Fear

Some people fear social judgment or embarrassment. They might avoid parties, work events, or even simple phone calls. This can limit their personal and professional life. Steps to address it include:

- **Gradual Social Steps**: Start with smaller gatherings or short interactions. Build up to larger events as you gain comfort.
- **Calm Self-Talk**: Replace thoughts like, "Everyone will think I'm silly," with, "Some people may not notice me much, and that's okay."
- **Focus on Others**: Shift attention to asking people questions or showing interest in them. This takes the spotlight off you and can lower anxiety.
- **Prepare Light Topics**: For large gatherings, think of a few simple topics to discuss, such as recent news or general hobbies. This can help avoid awkward silences.

Fear of Failure or Mistakes

Many people have a strong fear of failing. This can cause them to avoid trying new tasks or to work to the point of burnout:

1. **Realistic Goals**
   Set goals that are challenging but reachable. If the goals are too huge, the fear of failing can paralyze you.
2. **Learn from Errors**
   When you make a mistake, try to see it as feedback. Ask, "What does this teach me for next time?" rather than, "This proves I'm not good enough."
3. **Think in Steps**
   Break a big job into smaller parts. That way, if one part does not go well, it does not feel like a total failure.
4. **Recall Past Successes**
   When fear flares up, list times you did well in similar tasks. This helps balance the mind's focus on the negative.

Fear of Losing Control

Some worry that they might lose control in public, act strangely, or even harm themselves or others. This fear can be very distressing:

- **Check Reality**: Remind yourself that having the thought of losing control is not the same as acting on it.
- **Focus on Facts**: Ask, "Have I truly lost control before?" In many cases, the answer is no, which can help reduce the fear.

- **Safe Person**: If possible, be around someone you trust when you face the situation that triggers this fear. Their presence can reassure you.

Physical Exercise Against Panic and Fear

Movement can help manage fears by releasing built-up tension. While we discussed exercise in a previous chapter, here are some extra points tied to panic and fear:

1. **Short Bursts**
   When fear spikes, sometimes doing 20 quick jumping jacks or a short jog can burn off the excess adrenaline, helping the body return to a calmer state.
2. **Regaining Control**
   Exercise can remind you that your body follows your commands. This sense of control can counter the helpless feeling in panic.
3. **Team Activities**
   If social fear is an issue, joining a mild group sport or class can help you get used to being around others in a structured, low-pressure setting.

Unexpected Triggers

Fear does not always come from obvious sources. Here are some lesser-known triggers:

1. **Certain Sounds or Smells**
   These can unconsciously remind you of past scary situations. Noticing this link can help you address it.
2. **Caffeine or Other Stimulants**
   These can raise heart rate and mimic panic signs, leading you to feel fear when there is no true threat.
3. **Overthinking Bodily Sensations**
   If you notice a slight twinge or ache and jump to the worst conclusion, your fear can shoot up. Learning to read bodily signals more calmly can prevent unneeded worry.

Calming the Body's Alarm

If you are prone to panic, daily habits that calm the alarm system can help:

- **Consistent Routines**: We have talked about the power of routines. Knowing what to expect each day can ease overall tension.
- **Deep Breathing Practice**: Practicing breath control for a few minutes daily, even when calm, makes it easier to use during panic.
- **Progressive Muscle Relaxation**: This involves tensing and relaxing each muscle group. Doing it regularly can lower your default tension level.
- **Nature Breaks**: Spending some time in a park or near greenery can reduce stress hormones. Even a short moment around plants can help the nervous system relax.

Addressing Avoidance

When you fear something, the natural reaction is to avoid it. But avoidance can lock in the fear. Each time you avoid the feared situation, you never gather evidence that you could handle it. Here is how to fight avoidance:

1. **Small Steps**
   Tackle a mild version of the situation first. For example, if you fear crowded stores, start by going at a quiet time. Gradually work up to busier times.
2. **Plan and Reflect**
   Before facing the fear, plan how you will respond if anxiety shows up. Afterward, note what went right. This builds confidence.
3. **Support System**
   Ask a friend to come along the first few times. Having support can make the situation less daunting. Gradually, you can do it alone.
4. **Celebrate Progress**
   Even if you only handle half the situation at first, that is still progress. Recognize small steps as valid successes.

When Fear Turns to Phobia

Sometimes, fear grows into a phobia that disrupts daily activities. For instance, if you refuse to leave the house because of fear of having a panic attack, or you skip key medical tests because of a fear of doctors. In such cases, professional help is important. Therapy, and sometimes medication, can assist in shifting these deep-seated fears.

Special Tips and "Golden Gems"

1. **Fear Ladder**
   Create a list of your feared situations from least scary to most scary. Then work on them in order, practicing relaxation and positive thinking at each step. This is a structured way to manage fear without jumping straight into the worst case.
2. **Name the Fear**
   Give your fear a simple name, like "the worry bully." When it appears, you can say, "The worry bully is talking again, but I do not have to listen to it." This silly approach can help distance you from the feeling.
3. **Card Statements**
   Write short, calming statements on small cards, such as "This feeling will pass" or "I've survived this before." Keep them in your wallet or purse. When panic flares, reading these statements can bring quick relief.
4. **Limit Information Overload**
   Constant scary news or too much focus on horror stories can feed fear. If you notice you are more anxious after reading certain sites or watching certain shows, consider reducing that content.
5. **Posture Check**
   Sometimes standing or sitting up straight can help the body feel more secure. Slouching can restrict breathing and add to tension.

Looking Out for Triggers Early

Try to notice your earliest signs of rising fear:

- A slight change in breathing?
- Sweaty palms?
- Heart beginning to pound?
- Feeling hot or cold suddenly?

If you catch these signs early, you can do a quick grounding exercise or use calm self-talk to stop a full-blown panic. Often, fear grows when left unchecked. Early intervention can mean a milder episode.

Self-Compassion

Fear can make people feel ashamed. They might think, "I'm weak," or "No one else is this afraid." This is not true. Many people face fears and panic. Being kind to yourself can reduce the extra stress caused by shame. Accept that you are someone who feels fear strongly, and that you are working on tools to handle it. Shame often leads to isolation, but self-compassion can open the door to seeking help and making real changes.

Help from Others

1. **Safe Person**
   Have someone you trust who understands your panic or fear. They can step in with calming words or practical help if you start to feel overwhelmed.
2. **Professional Guidance**
   A counselor or therapist can provide tailored techniques for your specific fears. They have worked with many others in similar situations, so they often have a range of solutions.
3. **Online Resources**
   Some websites or support forums focus on panic and fear. Reading about others' progress can inspire you. However, be cautious of negative or inaccurate advice. Pick reputable sources, like mental health organization sites.

Progress Takes Time

Panic and deep fears rarely vanish overnight. Improving your response to them can be a gradual path. You might have setbacks. One day, you feel you have a fear under control. Another day, it suddenly appears stronger. That does not mean you failed. It is part of the process. Each time you use a coping skill, you strengthen your ability to handle fear. Over weeks or months, you may notice your panic episodes are less frequent or less intense.

Warning Signs of More Severe Issues

If panic or fear leads you to thoughts of harming yourself or if you feel you cannot function at all, please reach out for immediate professional help. This is not something to handle alone. There are crisis hotlines and mental health professionals trained to guide people through the darkest moments.

Linking Panic Management with Other Chapters

All the skills we have covered—like balanced routines, good self-talk, and stress management—make handling panic easier. For example, if you are well-rested, you might notice panic signs sooner and have the energy to apply your coping tools. If you have a supportive routine, you have anchors that reduce overall stress. Each piece supports the others.

Creating a Panic Plan

A panic plan is a short, clear outline of what to do if you sense a panic attack coming:

1. **Recognition**: "I know this is a panic sign. My heart is racing, but that does not mean I am in real danger."
2. **Calm Action**: "I will breathe in for four counts, out for four counts. I will do this five times."
3. **Grounding or Reassuring Statement**: "I am safe right now. This will pass."
4. **Seek Help if Needed**: "If this continues, I will step outside or call my friend for a quick chat."

Write it down. Keep it where you can see it. When panic hits, it can be hard to think clearly. Having a plan prepared can be life-changing in that moment of intense fear.

Looking Ahead

Panic and fear may be strong, but they are not unbeatable. By understanding how they work, you can use targeted techniques to reduce their hold on your life. Whether you face sudden panic attacks or long-standing fears, tools like slow breathing, grounding, and exposure practice can help. Over time, many people find these fears lose some of their force, allowing them to do things they once avoided.

In the next chapters, we will cover more topics that help complete the picture of managing anxiety. We will look at social anxiety, anxiety in work or school settings, mindset changes, and other specific challenges. Each chapter adds another layer to your toolkit, so you can handle different forms of worry and keep growing stronger. Panic and fear might still appear, but with each new skill, you become more prepared to face them and move forward with your goals.

Keep in mind that you are not alone in dealing with fear. Many people have felt their hearts pound or their stomachs twist at the thought of a dreaded situation. Yet many have found relief through steady practice of these methods. With patience and the right steps, you can reduce the power panic once had over you, and shape a life with more security and calm.

CHAPTER 11: SOCIAL ANXIETY

Social anxiety involves a strong fear of being judged or embarrassed when dealing with people. This anxiety can appear in many situations, such as parties, group events, or even casual chats. People with social anxiety might worry that others will think badly of them. They might avoid speaking up in class, skip gatherings, or say very little in group discussions. Over time, social anxiety can limit work, school, friendships, and daily life. In this chapter, we will look at what social anxiety is, how it forms, and ways to ease it. We will also share some lesser-known tips to help you feel more at ease in social settings.

What Is Social Anxiety?

Social anxiety is the feeling of stress or fear before, during, or after social situations. A person with social anxiety might feel tense when meeting new people, making phone calls, or attending parties. Some think that social anxiety is just shyness, but it can go beyond that. Shyness is a general personality trait. Social anxiety can include a deep fear of embarrassing oneself or being judged. This often leads to avoidance of many events or activities that could be fun or helpful.

While feeling a bit uneasy in new social settings is normal, social anxiety turns into a problem when it is strong and regular enough to keep someone from living normally. For example, a student might skip classes because they fear having to speak in front of classmates. An employee might refuse to give a short report at a team meeting. Over time, this can slow personal growth and block social connections.

Signs and Effects

1. **Physical Symptoms**
    - Racing heart
    - Sweating palms
    - Shaking
    - Dry mouth
    - Blushing

- Stomach upset
2. **Thoughts**
    - "Everyone is looking at me."
    - "What if I sound silly?"
    - "They will think I am boring."
    - "I will make a mistake and they will laugh."
3. **Avoidance Behaviors**
    - Skipping social gatherings
    - Eating alone to avoid talking to others
    - Not answering phone calls or messages
    - Avoiding eye contact or keeping conversations very short
4. **After Social Events**
   Many with social anxiety replay events in their head, picking apart every little thing they said or did. They might think, "I shouldn't have said that," or "They seemed annoyed with me." This can keep anxiety high, even after the event is over.

These thoughts and behaviors can cause a sense of loneliness, because avoiding people leads to fewer relationships. Work or school performance can suffer, because group projects or presentations might be too scary. Over time, self-esteem might drop, making the anxiety worse.

How Social Anxiety Develops

1. **Family Background**: If someone grows up in a household where social situations are seen as threatening, they might learn to be fearful. Hearing constant warnings such as "Watch out or they will make fun of you" can plant the idea that social events are risky.
2. **Bad Experiences**: If a person has faced bullying or harsh criticism, they might link social situations with shame or hurt. This can lead them to expect negative outcomes each time they talk to others.
3. **Personality Factors**: Some people have a natural tendency to be more sensitive. They might notice small social signals that others miss. This sensitivity can be helpful, but it can also mean they pick up on possible rejections or judgments more strongly.
4. **Social Media**: While it can help connect people, social media can also increase social anxiety. Seeing pictures of others having fun might make a

person fear they do not measure up. Or reading harsh comments online might fuel the worry of being judged.

Different Social Settings

Social anxiety does not look the same for everyone. Here are some common settings where anxiety can show up:

1. **Large Gatherings**: Parties or conferences can feel overwhelming because there are many unknown people.
2. **One-on-One Interactions**: Some find big groups easier, but fear small talk with one person. It can feel too personal and intense.
3. **Performance Situations**: Speaking up in a meeting, giving a speech, or performing in front of others can trigger anxiety.
4. **Online Settings**: Some people feel anxious sending messages or comments, because they fear negative reactions or being misunderstood.

Lesser-Known Factors in Social Anxiety

- **Facial Expressions**: Some people with social anxiety closely watch the faces of others, looking for signs of disapproval. They might see a tiny frown and think it is about them, even if the other person is just thinking of something else.
- **Mind Reading**: Believing you can guess what others are thinking, and of course assuming it is something negative.
- **Over-Preparation**: Spending hours scripting what you will say in every possible scenario can lead to more anxiety if the conversation goes off-script.
- **Leaving Early**: Some leave social events as soon as they arrive, feeling relief in the moment, but missing out on the chance to adapt to the situation.

Tips for Handling Social Anxiety

1. Gradual Exposure

Gradual exposure means you face social situations in small steps. Instead of jumping into a big party, start with inviting one friend for coffee. Then try a small group of friends. Over time, you build confidence and see that the feared outcomes (like extreme embarrassment) usually do not happen. This approach can change how your mind sees social events.

2. Balanced Thoughts

When you catch yourself thinking, "I will fail at this conversation," ask, "Is there solid proof I will fail?" Often, these thoughts are guesses, not facts. If you remind yourself that you have had normal talks before, you can challenge the fear that "this time will be a disaster." Balanced thinking might sound like, "I might feel nervous, but I can still talk normally."

3. Breathing Methods

Short breathing exercises before or during a social event can lower the body's alarm response. Try inhaling for a slow count of four, hold briefly, then exhale for four. Repeat a few times. This can calm the heart rate and reduce shaky feelings.

4. Focus on the Other Person

Social anxiety often comes from too much self-focus: "How do I look? Did I say something dumb?" Instead, place attention on the person you are talking to. Ask them questions, listen to their answers. This shift can reduce the loop of self-judgment in your mind.

5. Practice Simple Skills

If you find it hard to start conversations, prepare a few basic openers. For example, comment on the environment: "This cafe has great music, don't you think?" Or ask about the other person's interests. Simple questions like, "How did you choose this field of study?" can open a relaxed conversation. Over time, you will grow more comfortable improvising.

Social Skills Training

Some people with social anxiety feel they lack the skills to hold a conversation. This might include difficulties reading facial cues or responding in a friendly way. Social skills training can help. You could:

- **Join a Practice Group**: Some therapy programs or community centers run groups where you can safely practice small talk or group discussions without fear of harsh criticism.
- **Role-Play with a Friend**: If you trust someone, you can pretend to be in certain situations (like asking a coworker for help). It feels awkward at first, but it can prepare you for real-world events.
- **Watch Friendly Interactions**: Notice how people greet each other, ask questions, or share stories. Copying simple patterns can help you feel more at ease.

Dealing with Criticism or Rejection

One of the worst fears in social anxiety is being criticized or rejected. While it feels terrible to face a negative comment, it does not have to wreck your sense of self:

1. **Not Everyone Has to Like You**
   It might sound harsh, but it is true that not everyone will connect with you. This goes both ways—you also do not like every single person you meet. Accepting this truth can reduce the pressure to please everyone.
2. **Feedback vs. Insults**
   Sometimes people give feedback, which might feel like criticism but can be helpful if taken constructively. An insult is different—it is meant to harm. You can learn to tell them apart. If it is a mean insult, you can remind yourself it is not a fact about you, but rather a sign of that person's harshness.
3. **Practice Calm Replies**
   If you receive a negative remark, you can respond calmly by saying something like, "I hear your opinion, but I feel differently." Or you can simply say, "Thanks for sharing," and move on. Not every criticism deserves a big reaction.
4. **Build Self-Worth**
   The stronger your sense of self, the less power a rude comment has over

you. Practice reminding yourself of your good qualities, or keep a small list of your strengths. Over time, random negativity from others will not sting as deeply.

Handling Social Media Anxiety

Social media is a common area of stress. You might worry that your posts are not clever enough, or that you do not get enough "likes." If scrolling through feeds makes you feel bad, consider:

- **Time Limits**: Set a timer or use an app to limit how long you spend on social media. Constant checking can add to stress.
- **Selective Following**: If certain accounts make you feel inadequate, unfollow or mute them. Stick to content that is positive or helpful.
- **Private Sharing**: If you fear public judgment, share pictures or thoughts with a small, trusted group instead of posting to a large audience.
- **Remember Curated Lives**: People often show only their best moments online. It is not a full picture of their day-to-day life.

Seeking Professional Help

If social anxiety is strong and regular methods do not help, professional help can be very useful:

- **Counseling**: A therapist can help uncover the roots of your social anxiety and teach you targeted skills to manage it.
- **Group Therapy**: This is a setting where you can practice social skills in a supported group environment. Everyone there is working on similar issues.
- **Medication**: In some situations, doctors might prescribe short-term or long-term medication to ease symptoms, especially if the anxiety is very strong. This is usually most helpful when combined with therapy or self-help strategies.

Challenging Negative Beliefs

Many with social anxiety have beliefs such as: "I'm boring," "I have nothing of value to share," or "Everyone will notice if I slip up." These are filters that shape how you see yourself. To challenge these beliefs:

1. **Gather Proof of the Opposite**
   Look for times you had a decent conversation or moments you contributed a good idea. Write them down.
2. **Ask a Friend**
   Sometimes, a trusted friend can help you see your positive points. If they say you are funny or caring, this might feel more real than if you say it to yourself. Keep their words in mind next time a negative belief tries to take over.
3. **Be Fair**
   Notice how you respond to other people's small slips. You likely do not judge them harshly. Remind yourself that most people will treat your small mistakes the same way—they might not even notice them.
4. **Practice Kind Self-Talk**
   Each time you catch a harsh self-view, replace it with a softer line: "I might be nervous, but I still deserve a chance to speak."

Realistic Social Goals

Set goals that fit your starting point. If you rarely talk to anyone, maybe your first goal is to greet one coworker per day. Once that feels doable, raise the bar slightly. If you jump straight to giving a speech in front of 100 people, you might feel overwhelmed. Break bigger aims into smaller steps:

- **Goal 1**: "Say hello to a colleague and ask how their weekend was."
- **Goal 2**: "Stay at a small social event for at least 30 minutes."
- **Goal 3**: "Volunteer a short comment in a team meeting."

Celebrate each milestone you reach. Over time, you can do more than you first thought possible.

Dealing with Uncomfortable Moments

Even with practice, awkward moments can happen. You might trip while walking across the room or forget someone's name. Instead of viewing these as disasters:

- **Laugh It Off**: If you trip, you can say, "Oops, clumsy me today!" People often appreciate light humor about small mishaps.
- **Stay Calm**: If you forget a name, say, "I'm sorry, please remind me of your name." It is a common thing that happens to everyone.
- **Give Yourself a Break**: The event usually moves on. Most people do not dwell on small social slip-ups. Notice if you are the only one still thinking about it hours later.

When Friends or Family Do Not Understand

Some people might not get what social anxiety feels like. They might say, "Just relax" or "Stop worrying." This can be unhelpful. You can:

- **Explain Briefly**: You might say, "I sometimes feel extreme stress in social situations, and it is not just simple nervousness."
- **Ask for Specific Support**: If you are going to a party, you could ask a friend to stay nearby for the first few minutes until you feel settled. Or you might ask them to introduce you to one or two people, so you do not have to break the ice alone.
- **Seek Others Who Share Your Feelings**: There might be local groups or online forums about social anxiety. Connecting with others who truly understand can help you feel less alone.

Special Cases: Work or Class Participation

Social anxiety often shows up at work or school, where you must speak up to share ideas or ask questions. Here are ideas to make it easier:

1. **Advance Preparation**
   If you know you have to speak in a meeting or give a brief presentation, prepare points in writing. Practice out loud a bit. This can lower fear of freezing up on the spot.

2. **Use Visual Aids**
   Sometimes, bringing a short slide deck or a small handout can help. That way, the attention is partly on the material, not just on you.
3. **Arrive Early**
   If a meeting starts at 9:00 a.m., get there a bit early so you can settle in. Feeling rushed can increase nerves.
4. **Small Contributions**
   If you are uneasy about a group discussion, start by adding one or two quick remarks. Over time, as you see that it is okay, you might say more.

Beyond Anxiety: Building Genuine Connections

The end goal of easing social anxiety is not just to "handle" social events, but also to form better connections with others. Here are a few notes:

- **Quality Over Quantity**: You do not need to be friends with everyone. A few close relationships can be just as fulfilling as a large circle of casual contacts.
- **Be Curious**: People generally like to talk about their interests. Showing genuine curiosity can help you bond faster than focusing on yourself.
- **Listen Well**: Good listening is a valuable skill. If you reflect back what someone says, they feel heard. This helps build trust.
- **Practice Self-Care**: Rest well, eat well, and keep your stress levels in check. A balanced body and mind make it easier to connect with others.

Progress Takes Time

As with other forms of anxiety, social anxiety does not fade instantly. It involves learning new ways to handle worries and stepping outside your comfort zone step by step. Sometimes, you will feel like you are moving backward if you have a bad day or an awkward moment. That is normal. Each attempt is a chance to learn. Over weeks and months, you might discover you can talk to people more freely, join events with less dread, and even enjoy meeting new faces.

Common Pitfalls

1. **Comparisons**
   Comparing yourself to confident-looking people can feed your insecurity. Remember, you do not know what they feel inside, and everyone has strengths and weaknesses.
2. **Perfect Interactions**
   Some want every chat to go perfectly, with no pauses or missteps. That is not realistic. Normal conversations can have breaks or small stumbles.
3. **All-or-Nothing Thinking**
   If one event goes poorly, you might think, "This means I am doomed socially." That is an extreme view. Each event is a learning chance, and one rough experience does not define all future ones.
4. **Avoiding All Social Media**
   For some, total avoidance might be helpful if social media triggers big anxiety. But for others, cutting it out fully might lead to isolation. Look for a healthy middle ground, like limiting usage or curating your feed.

Putting It All Together

Social anxiety can feel like a big block, stopping you from enjoying life with friends or classmates. But many steps can reduce its power: balancing thoughts, practicing small chats, doing calming exercises, and seeking professional support if needed. With time, you can face social settings with more calm and less dread. You might even find that you enjoy certain events once the heavy fear fades.

This progress is usually slow but steady. Start with situations that feel only slightly scary and build from there. Track your wins, even if they seem small. Over weeks or months, you can look back and see how far you have come. You may find yourself able to speak up in groups, hang out with new people, or share your views without that pounding sense of panic. Each step forward boosts your confidence.

CHAPTER 12: ANXIETY AT WORK AND SCHOOL

Work and school are major parts of many people's lives. They can be places of growth, learning, and connection. However, they can also be sources of strong anxiety. Deadlines, performance reviews, tests, and group projects can create pressure. In this chapter, we will explore ways to reduce anxiety in these settings. We will discuss practical tips, from basic time management to lesser-known strategies, so that you can handle work or school challenges with more confidence.

Why Anxiety Appears at Work or School

1. **Performance Pressure**
   Many jobs and classes require good results. This might be meeting sales goals, finishing projects on time, or earning high grades. The fear of failing or losing a job can increase anxiety.
2. **Excessive Workload**
   Some workplaces and schools assign heavy tasks with strict deadlines. If you have too much on your plate, you might feel stressed about not finishing on time.
3. **Social Interactions**
   Work and school involve interacting with supervisors, coworkers, teachers, or classmates. If you have social anxiety, these daily interactions might feel tense or scary.
4. **Big Transitions**
   Starting a new job, moving from middle school to high school, or entering college can be stressful. A lot changes quickly, and uncertainty can fuel worries.
5. **Unclear Expectations**
   When instructions are not clear, you might worry about doing things wrong. If you do not know what a boss or teacher expects, you can feel nervous.

Effects of Anxiety on Work or School Performance

- **Trouble Concentrating**: Worries distract the mind, making it hard to focus on tasks or lectures.
- **Procrastination**: Anxiety can lead to putting off tasks because you fear failing.
- **Burnout**: Working or studying too long without proper breaks can lead to exhaustion, making anxiety worse.
- **Overthinking**: Spending extra time on small details instead of finishing assignments on time.
- **Avoidance**: Dodging group meetings, avoiding presentations, or skipping classes can become a pattern.

Time Management Skills

Managing time well can lower anxiety:

1. **Break Tasks into Steps**
   If you have a large project, list all the smaller parts. For a work report, this might mean: research, outline, writing, revising. For a school paper, it might be: choose topic, gather sources, draft, edit. Each step feels more doable.
2. **Set Priorities**
   Identify tasks that are most urgent or important. This ensures you do not spend too much time on minor tasks while ignoring big ones.
3. **Use a Planner or App**
   Writing down deadlines or using a scheduling app can help you avoid the fear of forgetting something. Check it each morning to plan your day.
4. **Realistic Scheduling**
   Do not pack your day with too many tasks. Leave some buffer time for breaks or unexpected delays. Trying to do everything at once can raise stress.
5. **Reward Yourself**
   After completing a major or tricky task, give yourself a small treat—maybe a short walk, a snack you enjoy, or a few minutes of a favorite pastime. This keeps motivation up.

Dealing with Deadlines

Deadlines can be a top source of anxiety. Here are ways to handle them better:

1. **Start Early**
   Even if you only do a small part of the task, starting early lowers last-minute panic. This also gives you room to revise if needed.
2. **Ask Questions**
   If a deadline seems too tight or the instructions are unclear, speak up. Talk to a boss, teacher, or classmate. Getting clarity can prevent wasted effort on the wrong approach.
3. **Draft First, Perfect Later**
   Sometimes, anxiety comes from trying to make the work perfect on the first attempt. Instead, do a rough draft or outline. Then you can improve it later.
4. **Track Progress**
   Note each small piece of the task you finish. This shows you are moving forward, which can calm the fear that you are stuck.
5. **Avoid Comparisons**
   Some people might complete tasks faster. That does not mean you have to. Focus on your own pace, as long as you meet the deadline.

Communication with Supervisors or Teachers

Open communication can lower anxiety at work or school:

1. **Clarify Expectations**
   If you do not fully grasp the instructions, ask for examples or confirm the main goals. Feeling certain about what is needed can reduce second-guessing.
2. **Check In**
   Periodically, let your supervisor or teacher know your progress. This can reassure them that you are on track and give you a chance to ask for any needed guidance.
3. **Request Extensions or Help Early**
   If you see a big obstacle, do not wait until the last minute to speak up. Many teachers or bosses appreciate an early heads-up so they can help you solve the problem.

4. **Stay Respectful**
   If you disagree with feedback, frame your response politely. For example, "I see your point. Could we discuss a different angle?" Polite communication often leads to helpful discussions.

Managing Test Anxiety

Students often face tests or exams, which can raise nerves. To reduce test anxiety:

1. **Prepare Properly**
   Cramming at the last minute can build fear. Spread out your study sessions, review notes daily, and quiz yourself.
2. **Healthy Study Environment**
   Find a quiet place where you can focus. Minimize phone notifications or loud music that can break concentration.
3. **Practice Under Real Conditions**
   Time yourself with sample tests. This helps you get used to the time pressure and lowers the fear of running out of time.
4. **Relax Before the Test**
   Do not study up to the very last second. Give yourself a few minutes to take deep breaths. Possibly do a quick stretch to release tension.
5. **Post-Test Review**
   If things go poorly, review what might have gone wrong. Maybe you needed more practice with certain types of questions. Learning from each test can reduce future anxiety.

Presentations and Public Speaking

Presentations can be nerve-racking, whether at school or in a job meeting:

1. **Plan Thoroughly**
   Have clear points or slides. Organize your ideas so they flow logically. If you know your material, you will feel more confident.
2. **Rehearse**
   Practice out loud, possibly in front of a mirror or with a friend. Time yourself. This helps you spot any confusing parts before the real event.

3. **Focus on the Message**
   Think about what you want the audience to learn or understand. Shifting attention from "they are judging me" to "they need this information" can reduce self-consciousness.
4. **Use Notes Wisely**
   Having small cue cards or an outline can be a safety net. Just do not read off them entirely—glance at them to stay on track.
5. **Positive Visualization**
   Picture yourself speaking calmly and finishing strong. While this alone may not cure stage fright, it can help keep your mind from only seeing worst-case scenarios.

Group Projects and Team Work

Group projects can cause anxiety if members have different work styles or if you fear conflict:

1. **Set Clear Roles**
   Early on, decide who does which part. Write it down so everyone knows their tasks. This reduces confusion and arguments later.
2. **Regular Check-Ins**
   Plan short team updates. For example, once a week. That way, if someone is falling behind, you can fix problems sooner.
3. **Communicate Respectfully**
   Even if you disagree with someone's approach, try to stay calm. Use phrases like, "I see your view, but could we look at it this way?" This avoids personal attacks.
4. **Ask for Help if Needed**
   If the group is stuck or a conflict is too big, contact the teacher or a supervisor. Delaying help might cause the project to fail.
5. **Celebrate Small Wins**
   When part of the project is done, acknowledge it. Positive feedback can keep everyone motivated and ease tension.

Workplace Conflicts

It is normal to have disagreements or misunderstandings with coworkers. Handling them well can lower anxiety:

1. **Direct Communication**
   If possible, speak privately with the person you have an issue with. Politely explain the problem. Ask for their side too. Clear talk often fixes issues before they grow.
2. **Stay Objective**
   Focus on actions or results, not personal traits. For example, "I noticed the report was not uploaded by Friday," instead of, "You are lazy and never do your work."
3. **Seek Mediation**
   If direct talk fails, involve a manager or human resources. They might help both sides find a fair solution.
4. **Know Your Boundaries**
   If a coworker is rude or crosses lines often, note it down. If it does not improve, you might need help from higher-ups.
5. **Self-Care**
   After a conflict, do something calming, like a short walk or a few deep breaths. Do not let the issue take over your whole day.

Online Meetings and Virtual Classes

With technology, many people work or study from home. This can also bring unique worries:

1. **Tech Setup**
   Make sure your internet, microphone, and camera are working before a meeting or class. Test them if you are unsure. Fear of tech issues can raise stress.
2. **Background Environment**
   If possible, find a quiet space. If you have to be in a shared area, let others know you have a meeting, or use headphones with a mic. This helps cut distractions.
3. **Eye Contact**
   Looking at the camera can simulate eye contact. If that feels too intense, look at the screen near the person's face. It still seems like you are engaged.
4. **Set Boundaries**
   Working or studying from home can blur lines between personal and

professional space. Try to stop work at a certain time, just as you would if you left an office or campus.

5. **Take Quick Breaks**
   Staring at a screen for hours can be draining. Block out short breaks to stand, stretch, or rest your eyes.

Handling Perfectionism

Both in school and work, perfectionism can lead to anxiety:

1. **Set Good-Enough Goals**
   It is fine to aim for quality, but recognize when a task is "good enough." Going beyond that point might not bring real benefits and can lead to missed deadlines.
2. **Accept Mistakes**
   Mistakes happen in learning and working. Many breakthroughs come from trying, failing, and adjusting. Fear of mistakes can freeze progress.
3. **Time Limits**
   If you spend too long polishing details, set a limit. Once the time is up, finalize and move on. This can prevent spirals of overthinking.
4. **Feedback**
   Ask a teacher or coworker what they expect. Sometimes you might assume they want a flawless masterpiece, but they might just need it done well enough to meet basic needs.
5. **Separate Self-Worth from Performance**
   Remind yourself that you are more than your job or grades. A poor result on a project does not define your entire value as a person.

Building Resilience

Resilience is the ability to bounce back from setbacks. In work or school settings, resilience helps you handle criticism, low grades, or negative feedback without feeling crushed:

1. **Learn from Each Struggle**
   Instead of thinking, "I messed up, so I'm a failure," try, "What can I do differently next time?" This shift helps you see challenges as lessons.

2. **Stay Flexible**
   Goals or deadlines can change. Being able to adapt your plan without panicking helps keep anxiety lower.
3. **Reach Out**
   If you are stuck, ask classmates, colleagues, or mentors for advice. You do not have to fix every problem alone.
4. **Celebrate Growth**
   When you handle a tough situation better than before, notice that progress. Positive reinforcement encourages further growth.

Health Habits for Better Performance

Taking care of your physical well-being can help lower anxiety at work or school:

1. **Hydration**
   Keep water on hand. Even mild dehydration can affect focus and mood.
2. **Balanced Meals**
   Eat foods that give sustained energy. Quick sugary snacks can lead to crashes, making you feel worse during a busy day.
3. **Short Activity**
   If you have a desk job or a long class schedule, do small movement breaks. A short walk or some gentle stretches can refresh your mind.
4. **Sleep**
   Lack of sleep reduces memory, focus, and emotional balance. Aim for a consistent bedtime, even during busy weeks.
5. **Screen Breaks**
   Looking at screens all day can strain your eyes and mind. Every hour or so, look away from the screen for a few seconds to let your eyes relax.

When to Seek Extra Help

Sometimes, work or school anxiety gets too big to handle alone. You might feel sick each morning, dread going to class or the office, or lose sleep all week. In such cases:

- **Counselors or Advisors**: Many schools have counseling services. Workplaces may have employee assistance programs. A short talk with a counselor can guide you toward effective strategies.

- **Support Groups**: Some communities or online platforms have groups for students with test anxiety or professionals feeling workplace stress. Talking with others in similar situations can reduce isolation.
- **Medical Input**: If anxiety leads to frequent headaches, stomach issues, or panic attacks, consider speaking with a doctor. They can check for any physical problems and suggest treatments, which may include medication if needed.

Handling Long-Term Career or Academic Anxiety

Anxiety can arise if you are unsure about your career path or major. You might think, "What if I picked the wrong field?" or "Will I find a good job after this program?"

1. **Research Options**
   Look into different career paths. Talk to people in those fields or set up informational interviews. Learning details can ease fear of the unknown.
2. **Get Guidance**
   Many schools have career centers that offer tests or counseling to match your interests with possible fields. At work, mentors or professional coaches can help you see paths for advancement.
3. **Try Small Steps**
   If you are unsure about a new direction, do a short volunteer opportunity or internship. This way, you get a feel for it before making a big change.
4. **Accept Adjustments**
   Many people switch majors or change jobs over time. An initial choice does not have to lock you in forever. Normalizing change can reduce anxiety about making a "wrong" choice now.

Lesser-Known Ideas for Work/School Anxiety

1. **Sound Therapy**
   Soft instrumental music or nature sounds can help some individuals focus while working or studying. Experiment with different options to see what helps you stay calm and productive.
2. **Desk Stretch Cards**
   Keep small cards with simple stretches at your desk or in your locker.

Every hour, pick a card and do a quick stretch to let go of built-up tension.
3. **Email Time Blocks**
   Constantly checking email or messages can raise stress. Set certain times to check your inbox, like mid-morning and mid-afternoon, so you can focus on tasks the rest of the time.
4. **Praise Jar**
   Keep a small jar or box where you drop notes about accomplishments. These can be tiny wins, like finishing a task early or helping a colleague. Reading them later can lift your mood when anxiety spikes.
5. **Visualization for Motivation**
   Rather than only picturing failure, try picturing yourself finishing a big project well or handing in a paper you are proud of. This can boost morale.

Balancing School/Work and Personal Life

It is easy to let work or classes take up all your time. That can lead to burnout. Try to set boundaries:

1. **End-of-Day Routine**
   Decide when you will stop working or studying each day (when possible). Put away materials, do a quick check of tomorrow's tasks, then switch to personal time.
2. **Plan Leisure**
   Schedule some fun or relaxing activities. This could be a hobby, a visit with friends, or time reading a fiction book. Having a break to look forward to can keep stress lower during the day.
3. **Unplug on Weekends**
   If your job or school schedule allows it, pick at least some weekend hours where you do not check work emails or assignments. This helps the mind recharge.
4. **Share Your Load**
   If you are overwhelmed, see if tasks can be delegated or if you can study with classmates for shared understanding. Trying to do it all alone can be a recipe for anxiety.

Tracking Your Growth

Just like in other areas of anxiety management, keep track of changes. For example:

- **Journal**: Write a short note each day or week about how stressed you felt at work or school. Record big events and how you handled them.
- **Look for Patterns**: Maybe you notice you are more anxious on days with certain tasks or classes. Adjust your approach based on these insights.
- **Celebrate**: When you handle a tough challenge or speak up in a meeting for the first time, acknowledge that success.

Over time, you might see that you are becoming more comfortable presenting ideas, meeting deadlines, and working with others.

Putting It All Together

Work and school can be stressful, but there are many tools to keep anxiety at lower levels. Time management, clear communication, and realistic goals can make a big difference. Regular breaks, supportive relationships, and a balanced routine can help you stay on track without feeling overloaded. If anxiety grows too large to handle alone, consider counseling or professional advice.

By applying these ideas, you can face tests, deadlines, and group tasks with more calm. It does not mean you will never feel nervous or stressed, but it does mean you will have ways to deal with those feelings without letting them ruin your performance or happiness. Over time, you can build skills that make you an effective student or employee, while also caring for your mental health.

The key is to start small. If you have a big project, break it down. If you worry about speaking up, begin with short comments. Each step forward can reduce fear and build confidence. As your confidence grows, you might find you actually enjoy certain tasks at work or school that once made you scared. Even if enjoyment does not come immediately, the fact that you can handle them without panic is a major win.

CHAPTER 13: MINDSET AND BEHAVIOR

Mindset and behavior play an important part in how people handle anxiety. Mindset is the way you think about yourself, your abilities, and your circumstances. Behavior is how you act based on those thoughts and beliefs. These two factors are linked. The way you think can guide your actions, and your actions can then shape how you see yourself and the world. When dealing with anxiety, adjusting both mindset and behavior can lower stress and give you a sense of control. In this chapter, we will explore specific ideas about mindset, how behavior patterns form, and practical ways to change them. We will also look at less-discussed facts and tips that you may find helpful.

Understanding Mindset

A "mindset" is a set of beliefs that determines how you see challenges. Some people have a "fixed mindset." They believe abilities and traits are set in stone: "I'm just not good at this, and I can't change." Others have a "growth mindset." They believe they can learn skills and develop traits over time: "I might not be good at this yet, but I can improve." While many people lean more to one side, you can shift your mindset on purpose. This can help manage anxiety because you see mistakes as learning points, not proof of failure.

Features of a Helpful Mindset:

1. **Openness**: Accepting that you do not know everything. Willing to learn new ways to handle stress.
2. **Self-Kindness**: Treating yourself like a friend instead of a harsh critic. This reduces shame and guilt.
3. **Curiosity**: Instead of quickly assuming the worst, you remain interested in what might happen. This can reduce fearful guessing.
4. **Adaptability**: Knowing life changes often and you can adjust rather than feeling helpless.

How Mindset Shapes Anxiety

- **Interpreting Events**: If you believe any bump in the road means total failure, you might feel anxious each time things do not go smoothly. A

flexible mindset allows you to see that mistakes are normal and not the end of the world.
- **Self-Esteem**: A harsh inner voice might say, "I always fail at everything." This lowers self-esteem and feeds anxiety about future tasks. A kinder view might say, "I am learning step by step," which leaves room for hope.
- **Resilience**: When you know you can learn and adapt, you become braver in facing problems. Anxiety may still show up, but you do not see it as proof of personal weakness.

Shifting to a More Helpful Mindset

1. **Spot Fixed Beliefs**: Write down strong statements like, "I can never handle social events" or "I am a weak person." Notice these as unhelpful beliefs.
2. **Question Them**: Ask, "Is it true I have never succeeded at a social event?" or "Am I always weak, or are there times I was strong?" Likely, you will see exceptions.
3. **Form New Statements**: Replace extreme thoughts with balanced alternatives. For example, "Social events are hard for me, but I have managed a few short gatherings. I can build on that."
4. **Practice**: Shift your mindset daily. Each time you catch a fixed belief, challenge it. Over time, your first thoughts become more open and less extreme.
5. **Gather Proof**: Notice small successes as evidence that you can improve. Perhaps you made a phone call you used to avoid. Jot it down as a sign of progress.

Behavior Patterns and Anxiety

Behavior patterns are repeated actions or choices you make. Some habits help reduce worry, like going for a daily walk or using a calm breathing technique when stressed. Other habits can increase anxiety, like avoiding certain tasks, staying up too late, or isolating yourself. Sometimes, people do not even see these habits forming. They just notice that they feel anxious.

1. **Avoidance**: One common pattern is avoiding anxiety triggers. For example, if you fear speaking up, you might skip all group discussions.

This brings relief in the short run but stops you from learning how to cope. Over time, the fear might grow.
2. **Perfectionism**: Another pattern is striving to make every detail flawless. This can lead to stress, missed deadlines, or constant self-criticism. The anxiety remains high because perfectionism is impossible to maintain.
3. **Self-Sabotage**: Sometimes, a person might wait until the last minute to do something because they are unconsciously afraid of failure. By causing a rush, they have an excuse if the outcome is not good.
4. **Overworking**: Trying to stay busy at all times to run away from anxious thoughts. Though it might bring a temporary distraction, overworking can lead to burnout and higher anxiety later.

Linking Mindset and Behavior

Your mindset tells you what is possible. If your mindset says, "I can't handle stress, so I must avoid it," you will likely avoid or delay things that cause anxiety. This short-term behavior might bring relief, but over time, it strengthens the mindset that you cannot deal with anxiety triggers.

On the other hand, if you adopt a more growth-oriented mindset—"I can learn to cope step by step"—you might take small actions to face challenges. Even if you do not succeed perfectly, each attempt helps you see that you can survive discomfort. This new evidence then builds an even more flexible mindset. Hence, changing either your mindset or your behavior can begin a positive cycle.

Action Steps to Adjust Behavior

1. **Create a Behavior List**: Write down one or two behaviors you want to reduce (like avoiding emails or procrastinating) and one or two you want to grow (like short daily workouts or reading for 10 minutes a day). Making this list visible can remind you of your aims.
2. **Use Gradual Goals**: If your avoidance is large, start with small steps. For instance, if you always avoid phone calls, your first step might be to answer one friendly call from a person you know well. Gradually, move to making short calls for appointments or information.

3. **Track Your Progress**: Keep a small notebook or app to mark days you practice the new behavior. Seeing streaks of success can be motivating, even if it is just a few days in a row.
4. **Reward Small Wins**: If you face a situation you usually avoid, give yourself a simple treat. This could be 15 minutes of a hobby you like, or a favorite snack. This helps your brain link the new behavior with a positive feeling.
5. **Plan for Slips**: Expect that sometimes you will fall back into old habits. This is normal. Do not see a slip as total failure. Instead, see it as a chance to learn what triggered it, and try again the next day.

Thought Replacement Techniques

Sometimes, anxious behavior is driven by automatic thoughts. Changing them in the moment can help you pick better actions:

- **Label the Thought**: When a negative thought appears, mentally label it as "just a thought, not a fact." For example, "I'll embarrass myself in this meeting" is a guess, not a certain truth.
- **Counter With Evidence**: Recall times you managed a similar situation. Write them down if needed. This evidence can weaken the anxious thought's hold.
- **Use Balanced Language**: Shift from "I will fail" to "I might feel nervous, but I can try my best, and it may turn out okay." This is neither blind positivity nor doom-filled thinking.

These steps do not remove anxiety instantly but give you a window of calm to choose a healthy behavior. Over time, your brain learns not to jump straight into panic mode.

Self-Observation

Watching how you act when anxious can reveal patterns. For a week, try this:

1. **When Anxiety Rises**: Note the situation (e.g., approaching a group, receiving a work email, etc.).
2. **How You Feel**: Quick words like "tense," "shaky," "worried," or "stomach tightness."

3. **Actions Taken**: Did you avoid the situation, try to numb yourself (maybe by scrolling on your phone), or face it directly?
4. **Outcome**: How did it end? Did you feel slightly better, or did it escalate? Did it teach you something?

This self-observation helps you spot which mindset or actions help and which make anxiety worse. It can also break the habit of reacting automatically. Even the act of writing things down can lessen the force of anxious thoughts.

Positive Behavior Experiments

Behavior experiments are a structured way to test negative predictions. If you think, "If I speak in this meeting, my boss will think I'm stupid," you set up a small test: plan one short comment or question in the meeting. Then see if your boss reacts badly or not. Often, you find that your worst fear does not come true. This evidence can chip away at your anxious mindset.

1. **Choose a Belief to Test**: For instance, "If I ask for help, people will reject me."
2. **Design a Small Action**: Ask a coworker for a small favor or ask a friend for advice on a minor issue.
3. **Observe the Response**: Did they reject you? Did they help? How did you feel?
4. **Record the Results**: Write down exactly what happened, avoiding guesses or distortions.
5. **Draw a Conclusion**: Does the original belief still stand? If not, replace it with a more accurate statement.

Repeating this method can reduce anxiety and reveal new possibilities.

Setting Boundaries for Healthier Behavior

One problem that fuels anxiety is the inability to say "no." People might say yes to extra tasks or social events out of fear or guilt. Later, they feel trapped and overwhelmed. Setting boundaries is a skill that ties mindset to action:

- **Identify Limits**: Figure out how much time or energy you can give without harming your well-being. This might be how many hours you can work, or how many social events you can attend in a week.

- **Practice Saying "No" Politely**: For example, "I appreciate the offer, but I don't have room in my schedule right now." This shows respect while protecting yourself.
- **Expect Discomfort**: It might feel awkward at first, but over time, saying "no" when needed reduces anxiety from overload. It also teaches others to respect your boundaries.

Building Self-Confidence Through Action

Sometimes, people wait to feel confident before attempting new behaviors. But often, confidence grows after the behavior. If you keep waiting for anxiety to vanish, you might never act. A better approach is:

1. **Start with Manageable Steps**: If you fear presenting in front of 20 people, try giving a short update to three colleagues first. Success in small steps can build confidence.
2. **Acknowledge Successes**: After each action, note what went well. Maybe you spoke clearly, or your heart rate dropped faster than usual. Focusing on small gains fosters confidence.
3. **Increase Complexity**: As small tasks become comfortable, slowly move to bigger tasks. This pattern of steady growth builds a record of capability.

The Role of Self-Talk in Behavior Change

Self-talk is the running commentary in your mind. When it is harsh—"I can't do anything right"—it can lead to avoidance or panic. Changing self-talk helps you take healthier actions:

- **Plan Specific Lines**: If you know you often get anxious before making phone calls, prepare a line like, "It's just a phone call, and I can handle it one step at a time." Repeat it before dialing.
- **Stop Catastrophic Thoughts**: If you catch yourself thinking, "This will be a complete disaster," say "Stop" in your mind, and replace it with a balanced statement. Over time, you will do this more naturally.
- **Give Credit**: After acting, say something like, "I did okay this time, and that's progress." This helps reinforce your new behavior.

Mindset Traps to Avoid

1. **All-or-Nothing Thinking**: Seeing any slip as total failure. This can sap motivation. Recognize that change is often uneven. One mistake is just one moment, not the end.
2. **Discounting the Positive**: Ignoring or downplaying small wins. If you do not see your successes, you stay stuck in a negative mindset.
3. **Labeling**: Using rigid labels like "I'm a coward" or "I'm useless." This blocks growth. Focus on specific behaviors instead of labeling your entire self.
4. **Emotional Reasoning**: Assuming that if you feel anxious, it must mean something awful is happening. Feelings can be real but are not always factual signals of danger.

Behavior Pitfalls to Watch For

1. **Substituting One Avoidance for Another**: You might quit one bad habit (like staying home from events) but adopt another (like escaping into social media). Check if you are just swapping ways to avoid stress.
2. **Overcomplicating**: Setting up a complicated system to handle anxiety can become another source of stress. Sometimes the simplest routines—like going for a 10-minute walk daily—are the best.
3. **Relying on Quick Fixes**: Certain substances or habits might numb worry temporarily, but they often lead to bigger problems. True change requires steady effort, not just temporary relief.

Group Support and Role Models

Sometimes, seeing other people who have faced anxiety and changed their mindset can inspire you. You could find these role models in:

- **Support Groups**: Online forums or in-person gatherings for people with anxiety. They might share how they switched from avoiding challenges to stepping forward.
- **Books or Interviews**: Reading stories of individuals who overcame big fears can give you insights for your own life.
- **Friends or Mentors**: A friend who bravely tried something new can motivate you to attempt your own step.

Observing how others talk about their struggles can help you adjust your own mindset. You might learn new behaviors or lines of self-talk that you never considered.

Using Affirmations Carefully

Affirmations are positive statements like, "I am strong and capable." Some people find them helpful, but others feel they are too forced, especially when anxiety is high. A balanced approach is to create affirmations that feel believable enough. For example:

- **Too Extreme**: "I will never be nervous again." (Likely false, leading to frustration.)
- **Balanced**: "I can face being nervous and still do what I need to do."

Use affirmations that acknowledge anxiety but do not let it stop you. This can gently shift your mindset without creating denial of real feelings.

Creating a Personal Growth Plan

Mindset and behavior changes do not happen by accident. A growth plan can guide you:

1. **List Key Areas**: Think about the top one or two areas where anxiety is highest. This might be social gatherings, public speaking, or dealing with conflict.
2. **Pick a Mindset Shift**: For example, if you fear social gatherings, shift from "I have to be perfect, or they will reject me" to "I can learn small steps to talk to people more comfortably."
3. **Pick One Behavior Change**: For that same situation, decide to attend a small gathering for 30 minutes. Prepare a few questions to ask someone. Keep it simple at first.
4. **Schedule Check-Ins**: Once a week, look at how you did. What worked? What was harder than expected? Did your anxiety go down or stay the same? Adjust your plan as needed.
5. **Add Over Time**: Once you feel some success, add another layer of challenge. Do not add too much at once. Growth is typically more stable when it is steady.

The Link Between Mindset, Behavior, and Physical Health

Taking care of your body can help with mindset and behavior changes:

- **Sleep**: Good sleep makes it easier to stay rational instead of panicking. A tired brain can revert to old anxious patterns more easily.
- **Nutrition**: Steady blood sugar can lower mood swings. If you skip meals or eat mostly sugary snacks, you might feel jittery, leading to negative self-talk or avoidance.
- **Physical Activity**: Regular movement can lower stress hormones in the body. This can help you feel calmer and more open to new actions.
- **Relaxation**: Practices like simple meditation or breathing drills can ground the mind, making it easier to notice self-defeating thoughts.

Motivation and Accountability

It can be easy to lose motivation when anxiety flares up. Some ways to stay on track include:

- **Buddy System**: Pair with a friend who has their own goals. Check in weekly. This can be as simple as texting each other your progress or having a short call.
- **Visual Reminders**: Put a sticky note on your desk with a short phrase that pushes you forward. Something like, "Small steps count" or "I am building new habits each day."
- **Professional Support**: Therapists or coaches can provide structure and cheer you on as you make slow but real changes.

Handling External Pressure

Sometimes, your environment can make mindset and behavior shifts harder. Maybe your family expects you to avoid certain topics, or your coworkers tease you for taking breaks. In these cases:

- **Explain Your Needs**: You can say, "I'm working on my anxiety levels, so I need to step out for a breath every so often."

- **Seek a More Supportive Environment**: If people around you constantly criticize your efforts, you might look for new social circles or at least limit time with negative influences.
- **Stay Firm**: Keep your boundaries. Change can be uncomfortable for others, especially if they were used to you acting differently. But your mental well-being comes first.

Checking Your Growth Over Time

Over weeks or months, you might see some of these signs:

1. **Less Avoidance**: Tasks or events that used to scare you become more approachable. You may still feel nerves, but you do not run away.
2. **Better Self-Talk**: You notice fewer harsh or extreme thoughts. When they do appear, you can counter them.
3. **More Tolerance for Discomfort**: Stressful moments do not feel as overwhelming. You might say, "This is tough, but I can get through it."
4. **Higher Self-Respect**: Each time you act in line with your new mindset, you prove to yourself that you can grow. This can result in deeper self-trust.

Overcoming Plateaus

Sometimes, progress stalls. You might feel stuck at a certain level of anxiety management. Strategies to move past plateaus include:

- **Try New Methods**: If you have been using only self-talk, consider adding behavior experiments or joining a support group.
- **Revisit Goals**: Perhaps the goals are too easy now, or too hard. Adjust them to your current level.
- **Get Feedback**: Talk to a mentor or therapist to see if they spot patterns you missed. Outside viewpoints can pinpoint hidden obstacles.
- **Refresh Your Motivation**: Remind yourself why you started changing your mindset. Think of the benefits—less worry, more freedom, improved relationships.

Practical Exercise: Daily Mindset Journal

A short, daily mindset journal can help maintain momentum:

- **Morning**: Write one belief you want to focus on, such as "I can handle unexpected problems calmly." Also note one new behavior you will try, like "I will approach a coworker and ask about their weekend."
- **Evening**: Note how the day went. Did you manage your mindset? What behavior did you try? Did it feel easy, hard, or in between? Any surprising results?

Over time, this builds a record of improvement, mistakes, and lessons. It also keeps you aware of your daily choices.

Moving Forward

Mindset and behavior are key pieces in handling anxiety. If you adjust how you see challenges and back it up with new habits, you create a lasting shift. This does not happen in one day. It requires steady, consistent effort. But each small action opens the door to bigger changes. You may find that tasks which once felt terrifying become only mildly uncomfortable, and eventually manageable. And that sense of progress can uplift your confidence in other areas of life.

Mindset shifts help you avoid seeing anxiety as a fixed destiny. Behavior changes help you live that new perspective in daily life. Taken together, they form a strong approach to mental health. You are not stuck with your current habits or beliefs. By noticing, questioning, and replacing them, you can shape a calmer, more balanced path.

In the next chapter, we will talk about long-term strategies. While daily tips and changes are important, we also need a bigger picture—ways to prevent relapse, keep growing, and handle new challenges that may appear over time. This next chapter will build on everything covered so far, helping you map out a future that is less weighed down by anxiety and more open to possibilities.

CHAPTER 14: LONG-TERM STRATEGIES

Short-term methods—like breathing drills or writing in a journal—can help you manage anxiety day by day. But real change often requires looking at the bigger picture. Long-term strategies aim to prevent anxiety from piling up again and to keep improvements going. This chapter will discuss ways to make lasting progress, maintain hope, and handle setbacks without losing ground. We will also cover some uncommon suggestions that might be valuable as part of a broader plan. By combining long-term thinking with the skills already learned, you can build a more secure base for steady well-being.

Why Long-Term Planning Matters

Anxiety often returns if we only rely on quick fixes or do not address underlying issues. For example, you might use a deep breathing method when tense, but if you keep living in a high-stress environment and never manage your workload or emotional triggers, anxiety can climb back. Long-term strategies help you:

1. **Build a Stable Lifestyle**: Setting boundaries, maintaining healthy routines, and getting the right support can prevent stress overload.
2. **Develop Mental Strength**: Over time, regular practice of coping skills makes them second nature, so you can handle bigger life changes.
3. **Maintain Motivation**: Knowing you have a plan for growth can keep you hopeful even when daily life is tough.

Setting a Vision for Your Well-Being

A helpful step is to decide on a long-term vision for how you want your life to look, especially regarding mental health. This vision might include:

- **Emotional Goals**: You might want to feel more calm on normal days, handle conflict better, or reduce negative self-talk.
- **Behavior Goals**: Perhaps you want to travel more, try a new hobby, or improve relationships without being held back by anxiety.
- **Life Goals**: Maybe you plan to pursue a new career path or further education once anxiety is under control.

This vision is not a strict rule. Rather, it is a guide. By having a clear picture of why you are working on anxiety, you keep your focus. When you face setbacks, recalling your overall goals can remind you why it is worth pushing on.

Physical and Mental Maintenance

Long-term strategies require consistency in these areas:

1. **Physical Health**: Continue to prioritize sleep, nutrition, and movement. An exhausted or nutritionally deprived body is more prone to anxious feelings. Think of these basics as daily fuel for your mind.
2. **Emotional Monitoring**: Check in with yourself from time to time. Ask, "How high is my stress level today?" or "Am I feeling more irritable than usual?" Early detection helps you act before a crisis.
3. **Regular Relaxation**: Make time each week for a calming activity. It could be art, music, nature walks, or a simple routine like a warm bath. Ongoing relaxation helps prevent tension from building up too much.

Strengthening Support Networks

Support is often key for long-term stability. It is easier to keep improvements going when you have people around who understand and respect your needs.

- **Family and Friends**: Share with them your goals regarding anxiety. Let them know how they can support you. This might be checking in, encouraging you to keep up a habit, or simply listening when you feel uneasy.
- **Peer Groups**: Find online or local groups of people working on similar challenges. These groups can offer fresh tips, empathy, and accountability.
- **Professionals**: Even if you have moved past a crisis point, occasional check-ins with a counselor or therapist can keep you on track. Think of it as preventive care for your mental health.

Updating Goals Over Time

As you grow, your needs and challenges might shift. A long-term plan is not static. It can be revised:

- **Annual or Semiannual Review**: Once or twice a year, sit down and see what has changed. Is your anxiety level lower in some areas but still high in others? Maybe you overcame social fear but now face work stress. Update your goals accordingly.
- **Celebrate Milestones**: When you see how far you have come, it builds confidence. If you used to fear making phone calls and now it is easy, note that progress and allow yourself to feel a sense of achievement.
- **Add New Challenges**: If you have mastered basic coping methods, consider adding more advanced tasks. This could be tackling a bigger fear or developing leadership skills at work once anxiety about speaking has faded.

Building Resilience to Stressful Events

Life has ups and downs. Even if you have made progress, a big event—a job loss, a personal loss, or unexpected changes—might cause new waves of anxiety. Long-term strategies include preparing for the unexpected:

- **Emergency Coping Kit**: Keep a list of phone numbers, calming exercises, or short reminders that have helped you in the past. When a crisis hits, it is harder to think clearly, so having a kit ready can be a lifesaver.
- **Financial and Practical Planning**: Money problems can fuel anxiety. Where possible, having a small savings buffer or a plan for emergencies can ease worry. Similarly, being organized with important documents can lower stress when life shifts suddenly.
- **Emotional Support System**: Identify one or two people you can reach out to if you feel overwhelmed. It might be a close friend, family member, or hotline. Knowing you have someone to call can reduce fear of facing problems alone.

Mindful Lifestyle Choices

Developing a mindful lifestyle means being aware of how your environment affects you. These are some elements to consider:

1. **Digital Boundaries**: Constant news feeds or social media can raise stress. Decide on specific times to go online. Turn off non-essential alerts. This can protect you from a stream of negative or distracting updates.
2. **Tidiness**: A messy living space can make it harder to relax. Simple tidying or organizing can give a sense of control and calm. This does not mean striving for perfection, just keeping your environment supportive.
3. **Scheduling Downtime**: If your calendar is full every day, you might never have a moment to decompress. Booking downtime—where you do nothing pressing—can prevent burnout and keep anxiety from building.

Balancing Work, Personal Life, and Rest

Long-term mental health often involves balanced living:

- **Work-Life Separation**: If possible, try not to bring work stress home all the time. Some people remove work email apps from personal devices or set firm cut-off times in the evening.
- **Hobbies**: Engaging in an activity you find interesting can relieve stress. Whether it is learning an instrument or trying a creative craft, hobbies can keep your mind active in a positive way.
- **Social Connections**: Healthy relationships can buffer against stress. A chat with a friend or a shared activity can ease anxious feelings. Make time for these connections, even if it is just a quick call once a week.

Updating Self-Talk and Thought Patterns

Anxiety can sometimes fade, but old thought habits might creep back if left unchecked. Long-term strategies should include continued attention to self-talk:

- **Regular "Thought Check"**: Every so often, ask yourself if your thoughts are veering toward extreme negativity again. If you catch these patterns early, you can correct them before they become ingrained.

- **Deepen Your Skills**: If you already learned how to replace negative thoughts, try more advanced techniques. For instance, you might learn about Acceptance and Commitment Therapy (ACT) or other structured methods that go beyond basic thought replacement.
- **Teach Others**: Helping a friend or family member with a thought-checking method can reinforce your own skills. Teaching often clarifies your knowledge.

Periodic Therapy or Counseling Tune-Ups

You do not need to be in crisis to benefit from talking with a counselor or therapist from time to time. These check-ups can help you:

1. **Spot Hidden Issues**: A professional might see small signs of old anxiety returning or find new concerns you have not noticed.
2. **Learn New Approaches**: Mental health research continues to grow. A therapist might share recent strategies or tools you have not tried yet.
3. **Stay Accountable**: Knowing you have a session scheduled can keep you motivated to maintain your mental health habits.

Planning for Future Growth

People often think anxiety management is just about removing fear. But many find that once they handle anxiety, they can add positive experiences. For example:

- **Career Growth**: You might aim for a promotion or start a side project that used to feel too scary.
- **Social Expansion**: You might join a club or community group because social fear has less hold now.
- **Personal Development**: You could learn new skills, like a language or cooking style, that once felt too intimidating.

Having a plan for positive growth ensures anxiety is not just absent, but replaced with fulfilling activities.

Handling Relapses or Setbacks

Even with strong progress, setbacks can happen. You might face a sudden spike of anxiety after a tough event or slip back into old habits during a stressful time. This does not mean your progress is lost:

1. **Recognize Temporary Upsets**: A relapse could be short if you address it early. Do not assume it will last forever.
2. **Return to Basics**: Use the core tools that helped you before. Maybe that is a daily relaxation practice, a short routine that balanced your mood, or a journaling habit.
3. **Seek Support**: If the setback feels bigger than you can handle alone, turn to a friend, group, or professional for a fresh boost.

Less-Discussed Long-Term Tools

1. **Biofeedback**: A technique where you use sensors to track heart rate or muscle tension, learning to calm them down in real time. Over many sessions, you might gain more control over your body's stress reactions.
2. **Volunteering**: Helping others can shift focus away from personal worries. Plus, it can give a sense of purpose. This is not to deny your own needs, but to create a healthier perspective.
3. **Creative Expression**: Writing poems, painting, or playing an instrument can allow you to release stored feelings. This does not require being "good" at these arts; the act itself can be soothing.
4. **Physical Challenges**: Activities like hiking, gentle martial arts, or even learning a new sport can build confidence. Meeting physical challenges can teach you that you can also handle mental challenges.

Lifestyle Choices That Support Long-Term Stability

1. **Limit Harmful Inputs**: If certain movies, shows, or news sources make you anxious for days, reduce them. This does not mean avoiding all negative topics, but being mindful of your limits.
2. **Spending Time in Nature**: Research suggests that time spent around trees or water can lower stress hormones. A simple weekly walk in a park might help long-term calm.

3. **Goal Refresh**: Every few months, adjust your personal and professional goals to keep them realistic. Goals that are too high or too vague can breed anxiety.

Building Inner Confidence Over Time

Confidence grows with practice and proof. The more you handle difficult moments, the more evidence you gather that you can cope. While it is helpful to aim for confidence, do not wait to act until you feel 100% sure. Action itself often triggers more trust in your abilities.

- **Collect Success Stories**: Keep a journal page dedicated to successes in dealing with anxiety. If you overcame a fear of public transport or managed a heated discussion calmly, write it down. Over time, this page will become a personal reminder of your growth.
- **Practice Calm Responses**: Mentally rehearse how you will respond to triggers. Whether it is an unplanned event or a social snub, having a mental script can reduce panic if it actually happens.
- **Adopt a Forward-Looking View**: Anxiety often centers on fear of what might happen. By focusing on each step you are taking toward a better future, you shift from worry to action.

Community Involvement

Long-term strategies are supported by involvement in positive communities. This can be:

- **Clubs or Classes**: Learning a skill with others builds social ties and new experiences, which can keep you from slipping into isolation.
- **Religious or Spiritual Groups**: If it fits your beliefs, belonging to a supportive spiritual community can provide comfort and a sense of belonging.
- **Local Advocacy**: Working on local causes or volunteering in community projects can give you a sense of purpose beyond your own anxieties.

Using Technology Wisely

While technology can cause distraction or stress, it can also aid long-term mental health:

1. **Mood-Tracking Apps**: Logging daily moods and triggers can help you see progress or identify patterns.
2. **Meditation Apps**: Some apps provide guided exercises for relaxation or mental focus, which can be part of your long-term plan.
3. **Online Counseling**: If in-person therapy is difficult due to distance or schedule, online sessions can offer flexibility.

Recognizing and Adjusting to Life Transitions

Life changes like moving, changing jobs, starting or ending relationships, or having children can trigger fresh anxiety. A long-term plan includes readiness to adapt:

- **Learn About the Next Step**: If you move to a new city, look up local groups or resources in advance. If you change jobs, read about the new company or role. Knowledge reduces fear of the unknown.
- **Maintain Old Coping Tools**: Even if a new environment feels different, the same breathing methods, self-talk, or journaling can still help.
- **Find Local Support**: In a new area, search for support communities or friendly acquaintances who can show you around or offer insight. This can reduce isolation quickly.

Keeping Hope Alive

Maintaining hope is crucial for long-term progress. Anxiety can cause people to think changes will not last or that problems will return. A few suggestions:

1. **Track Even Tiny Improvements**: Over weeks or months, a small improvement here or there can add up. Recognizing these helps you see you are always moving forward.

2. **Practice Gratitude**: This does not mean ignoring real problems. However, noticing good things—like a helpful friend or a sunny day—can balance out worry-focused thinking.
3. **Look at Role Models**: Others have faced serious anxiety and found lasting ways to live more peacefully. Reading or hearing their stories can confirm that long-term improvement is possible for you too.

Putting It All Together for the Future

Your long-term plan might include daily habits (like short movement sessions or calm breathing), weekly check-ins (such as journaling or group meetings), and periodic reviews (to see how far you have come and where you can grow). As new challenges appear in life, you can fold them into your plan, adjusting your goals and methods. In this way, you build a lifestyle that supports lower anxiety rather than a one-time "fix."

Long-term strategies do not remove all worry from life. Some anxiety is natural. But they do keep worry from overpowering you at every turn. They help you form a stable ground so you can move toward your aspirations with more confidence. Over time, this steady approach can transform anxiety from a huge stumbling block into a smaller hurdle you can handle. It might still show up, but you will have the tools and mindset to address it.

With a good long-term framework, each new day can be one of practice and growth, instead of dread. You do not have to feel perfect to make progress. You just need to stay open to learning, keep an eye on your habits, and adapt your plan to the realities of your life. As you do so, you build a deep reservoir of coping skills. When stress rises, you can tap into that reservoir, trusting that you have faced difficulties before and come out stronger. That sense of trust in yourself is one of the greatest rewards of a long-term commitment to handling anxiety.

In the chapters to come, we will look at more ways to address anxiety from different angles, including medication and therapy options, breaking harmful habits, and finding strength in the face of uncertainty. Each piece fits into the larger puzzle of mental health. By combining daily tactics with big-picture thinking, you can nurture a stable and lasting sense of calm, even in a changing world.

CHAPTER 15: MEDICATION AND THERAPY

Medication and therapy can both play a part in helping people handle anxiety. They do not always work for everyone in the same way, but many find these tools useful. In this chapter, we will talk about different kinds of medication, basic therapy options, how to know if these approaches might help, and simple facts that many people do not know. The focus is on providing clear, easy-to-follow information so you can make well-informed decisions.

Why Consider Medication or Therapy?

Some people can manage anxiety with practical steps alone, such as relaxation or changing their routine. But there are times when anxiety is deep, causing panic attacks or serious trouble with daily tasks. When it gets in the way of work, school, or having normal conversations, it might be time to think about extra support.

Medication can calm the body's alarm system, making anxious feelings less intense. Therapy can teach strategies to handle worry, fear, or negative thoughts. Sometimes using both together helps. These are tools you can explore if day-to-day tactics do not lower anxiety enough.

Different Types of Medication

Medications for anxiety often fit into certain groups. While the exact name or brand can differ, most belong to one of these categories:

1. **SSRIs (Selective Serotonin Reuptake Inhibitors)**
    - Examples: drugs often made to help with depression, but they can help anxiety too.
    - How They Work: These raise serotonin levels in the brain. Serotonin is linked to mood. When levels are more balanced, anxiety might drop.
    - Things to Know: It can take a few weeks before a person notices less anxiety. Sometimes there are side effects, like feeling restless or having stomach issues, but these often lessen over time.

2. **SNRIs (Serotonin-Norepinephrine Reuptake Inhibitors)**
   - Examples: another set of meds used for depression and anxiety.
   - How They Work: They help both serotonin and norepinephrine. Norepinephrine can affect energy and focus. Balancing these might reduce worry.
   - Things to Know: Similar to SSRIs, it can take a few weeks to see big changes. Possible side effects might include mild sleep problems or a headache, but many people adjust.
3. **Benzodiazepines**
   - Examples: sometimes used for short-term relief of strong anxiety or panic.
   - How They Work: They slow down some brain activity, creating a calming effect. This can be quick, which is why they are sometimes used in emergencies.
   - Things to Know: These can be habit-forming if used for a long time. Health professionals often suggest them for short periods or specific cases, rather than as a long-term fix.
4. **Beta-Blockers**
   - Examples: originally made for heart issues, but can help with physical signs of anxiety, like a racing heart.
   - How They Work: They block certain stress hormones, keeping heart rate and shaking down.
   - Things to Know: They do not always change negative thoughts, but they can help in situations like public speaking by reducing fast heartbeat and trembling.
5. **Other Options**
   - A health professional might suggest other meds if a person's anxiety has special factors. Some older types of medication still help certain people, but SSRIs and SNRIs are common first choices. Others might consider natural or over-the-counter products, but these can vary a lot, and it is wise to check with a qualified person to see if they are safe.

What to Expect with Medication

- **Starting Up**: Some medication takes time to adjust. A person might have mild side effects like feeling more sleepy, slight nausea, or changes in

appetite. These often lessen in a few weeks, but if they are severe or do not go away, talking to a health professional is important.
- **Finding the Right Dose**: It is normal to begin with a lower dose and raise it slowly. This helps the body get used to it. Jumping too high too fast can worsen side effects.
- **Sticking with It**: If a medication helps, some people might take it for months or a year or more. Others might stay on it longer if anxiety returns each time they stop. There is no single rule for everyone.
- **Going Off Safely**: If a person decides to stop, it is best to do so under guidance from a health professional, who can create a plan to avoid withdrawal.

Myths About Medication

1. **Myth: Medication Changes Who You Are**
   Fact: It does not turn a person into someone else. It can help calm overwhelming signs of anxiety, giving a clearer mind to handle daily life.
2. **Myth: Only Weak People Take Medication**
   Fact: It is a tool. Just like using a cast for a broken bone, medication can assist with healing or management.
3. **Myth: All Medications Are Addictive**
   Fact: Some types can create dependence if used too long (like certain benzodiazepines), but SSRIs and SNRIs are not known to be addictive in that way.
4. **Myth: Once You Start, You Cannot Stop**
   Fact: Many people use medication for a certain period, then slowly reduce or stop with guidance. They might use therapy or lifestyle changes to stay stable.

Therapy Approaches

Therapy can teach ways to handle anxious thoughts and habits. It can also help uncover the reasons behind worry. Different therapy styles exist, so finding a good match is key.

1. **Cognitive Behavioral Therapy (CBT)**
   - Focus: Changing negative thoughts and behaviors.

- Methods: The person and therapist work together to spot harmful thinking patterns and replace them with more balanced ones. They might also use step-by-step exposure to fears.
- Why It Helps: CBT offers specific tools and homework, so changes can happen between sessions too. Over time, repeated practice can shrink anxiety.

2. **Dialectical Behavior Therapy (DBT)**
    - Focus: Handling intense emotions and building strong coping skills.
    - Methods: Uses mindfulness, managing feelings, and balancing two things at once: accepting the current moment but also working on change.
    - Why It Helps: It can be especially useful if anxiety is tied to big mood swings or if a person feels overwhelmed by strong emotions.

3. **Acceptance-Based Methods**
    - Focus: Learning to notice and accept anxious feelings without letting them control behavior.
    - Methods: Might involve exercises that let a person observe thoughts and feelings calmly, plus making choices aligned with personal goals.
    - Why It Helps: Some anxiety grows when trying to fight or push away every worry. Accepting it can reduce its power.

4. **Exposure Therapy**
    - Focus: Gradually facing the things that cause fear.
    - Methods: A step-by-step approach where the person starts with less scary tasks and moves to bigger ones. Over time, the mind learns that the fear can be managed.
    - Why It Helps: Repeated safe exposure shows the brain that danger is less than it thinks. This helps reduce panic in real-life situations.

5. **Group Therapy**
    - Focus: Sharing experiences with others who have similar worries.
    - Methods: A trained leader guides discussions and exercises. Group members give feedback or support each other.
    - Why It Helps: Realizing you are not alone can lower shame. Watching how others handle anxiety can give ideas for your own situation.

What Happens in a Therapy Session?

While therapy sessions vary, a typical session might include:

- **Check-In**: The person shares how they have been feeling since the last meeting.
- **Review of Past Actions**: If there was homework or a plan, they talk about what worked and what did not.
- **New Skills**: The therapist might teach a new technique or help the person see how to handle a specific problem.
- **Discussion**: They might talk about deep topics or practice new behaviors.
- **Plan**: They agree on tasks or goals to work on before the next session.

Therapy is not just about talking; it usually involves trying out skills in real life. It can also be short-term or long-term, depending on need.

Combining Medication and Therapy

Some people find the best results when they use both medication and therapy. Medication might calm strong anxiety signs, making it easier to focus on therapy tasks. Therapy can then help a person build skills that last beyond the time they might need medication.

1. **Short-Term vs. Long-Term**: Some use medication for a short while to get anxiety under control, then rely more on therapy or lifestyle changes. Others might keep taking medication if signs return without it.
2. **Adjusting Doses**: A health professional might raise or lower medication doses as therapy progresses and the person learns new skills. This requires check-ins to see how everything is working together.
3. **Communication**: If different professionals are involved—like a doctor for medication and a therapist for sessions—it helps if they can share updates (with your permission). This way, all parts of the plan align.

Finding the Right Professional

1. **Doctors or Psychiatrists**: They can prescribe medication and monitor physical health. Some also do therapy, but many focus on diagnosing and managing meds.

2. **Counselors or Therapists**: They provide various types of therapy but do not usually prescribe medication. They might have degrees in psychology or social work.
3. **Questions to Ask**:
    - "Do you have experience treating anxiety?"
    - "What methods do you use?"
    - "How often do you suggest sessions?"
    - "What costs are involved?"
    - "Do you accept insurance, or is there a sliding scale for fees?"

It might take a few tries to find a good fit. If you do not feel comfortable after some sessions, seeking another option can be wise. A strong relationship with the professional is important for progress.

Getting the Most Out of Therapy

- **Regular Attendance**: Missing sessions often can slow progress.
- **Open Communication**: If something is not helping or if you feel worse after a session, tell the therapist. They might adjust the approach.
- **Homework Practice**: Many therapy methods include tasks between meetings, like writing in a journal or trying a new behavior. Doing these is key to lasting improvements.
- **Patience**: Therapy can help quickly sometimes, but deeper changes often need time. Some people see small shifts in a few weeks, but bigger ones in a few months.

Special Settings: Teletherapy and Online Help

Some people cannot go to an office due to distance or schedules. Online therapy can be an option. It uses video calls, phone calls, or chats. While it might feel different from face-to-face contact, many find it effective for anxiety. It is important to check that the service is professional and follows privacy rules.

Lesser-Known Therapy Ideas

1. **Art or Music Therapy**: Using creative projects to express feelings. This can help people who find it tough to explain thoughts in normal conversation.
2. **Animal-Assisted Therapy**: Spending time with trained animals like dogs or horses can help a person relax. This is not a fit for everyone, but some see calming effects.
3. **Sensorimotor Therapies**: Methods that focus on how the body stores feelings. They can include small movements or noticing posture and muscle tension to help release anxiety.
4. **Brief Therapies**: Some approaches focus on short, structured sessions to target a specific problem. They can be a good fit if you have a clear goal, like conquering fear of flying.

Warnings and Safeguards

- **Unsafe Claims**: Watch out for anyone who claims to fix anxiety instantly or says their single product can solve all problems. Anxiety is complex, and real progress usually takes more than one method.
- **Medication Interactions**: If you take other medicines (for blood pressure or other conditions), always let the doctor or therapist know so they can check for conflicts.
- **Therapy Boundaries**: A good therapist keeps the discussion professional. If you feel unsafe or pressured, it is okay to switch to another therapist.
- **Time Frames**: Each person's body and mind differ. One might notice changes in a couple of weeks, while another might need months. There is no shame in going slower than others.

Golden Tips for Medication and Therapy

1. **Track Your Symptoms**: Writing down daily anxiety levels, side effects, or improvements helps you see patterns. This record can guide your professional to adjust the plan more accurately.
2. **Ask Questions**: Whether it is about side effects, therapy homework, or how the approach works, asking questions can give you peace of mind.

3. **Combine with Healthy Living**: Even if medication lowers anxiety, unhealthy habits (like poor sleep or too much caffeine) can keep levels high. Good sleep, balanced meals, gentle exercise, and therapy usually work better as a complete plan.
4. **Stick to a Schedule**: For meds, take them at about the same time each day to keep levels steady. For therapy, keep appointments consistent, so momentum is not lost.
5. **Avoid Abrupt Changes**: Stopping medication quickly can cause unpleasant effects. Shifting therapy methods too often can slow progress. Slow, planned changes are safer.

Personalizing Your Approach

Medication and therapy options are personal. Some may do well with a low dose of an SSRI for several months and weekly CBT sessions. Someone else might choose no medication but do intense exposure therapy. Another might switch approaches after realizing the first method was not helping enough. None of these paths are "wrong." It is about finding what fits your body, mind, and life.

Moving Ahead

If your anxiety stops you from living fully, it can help to consider medication or therapy. These tools are not magic solutions, but many people see less worry, better focus, and renewed hope. By mixing daily habits—like healthy routines, supportive mindsets, and taking breaks—along with medication or therapy if needed, you create a more complete strategy to handle anxiety. You do not have to face it alone. With the help of skilled professionals and simple self-care practices, you can feel steadier, more able to enjoy each day.

In the next chapter, we will talk about breaking harmful habits. While medication and therapy can be strong aids, sometimes our own daily choices add to the problem. We might overuse certain substances or behaviors that raise worry. Identifying and dropping these habits can work together with medication and therapy. The aim is to remove extra hurdles so that progress is smoother and more permanent.

CHAPTER 16: BREAKING HARMFUL HABITS

People often develop habits that reduce anxiety for a moment but cause more problems later. These habits might be tied to substances, behaviors, or thought patterns. Over time, they can worsen worry and keep you from building healthier ways to cope. This chapter looks at common harmful habits, why they form, and how to stop them. We will also share practical tactics and less-common facts that can help break these patterns for good.

What Are Harmful Habits?

A harmful habit is an action done repeatedly that hurts mental or physical health. Some examples include:

1. **Excessive Alcohol or Substance Use**: Using alcohol, nicotine, or drugs to calm nerves can lead to addiction, health issues, and more anxiety when the substance wears off.
2. **Misuse of Food**: Some people turn to overeating sugary or fatty foods for comfort, while others do not eat enough. Both can affect mood and body health.
3. **Too Much Screen Time**: Hours of scrolling through social media or playing online games can push you to ignore real stress, leaving it unresolved.
4. **Avoiding Responsibilities**: Putting off tasks until the last minute can give short relief, but the stress piles up.
5. **Negative Mental Loops**: Constantly predicting worst outcomes or calling yourself names can become a habit too, making it tough to see hope.

Why Do We Develop These Habits?

- **Instant Relief**: Drinking, smoking, or browsing the internet might bring short-term relief from anxious feelings. Our brains can get used to that quick fix.
- **Social Pressure**: Friends or family might do the same thing, and we join in without much thought. Over time, it becomes a habit.

- **Lack of Other Tools**: If a person does not know healthy ways to handle anxiety, they might turn to whatever offers even a little relief.
- **Brain Chemistry**: Certain habits, especially those involving addictive substances, can change the brain's reward system. This makes quitting feel harder because the body craves the substance or action.

How Harmful Habits Increase Anxiety

1. **Physical Toll**: For instance, too much caffeine can cause jitters, racing heart, or trouble sleeping, which can mimic anxiety signs. The same goes for sugar crashes.
2. **Emotional Cycles**: A person might feel guilty or ashamed after indulging in a habit. This negative feeling can trigger even more anxiety, leading them to repeat the habit for relief.
3. **Avoidance Grows**: If you use these habits to run from stress, you never face the real problem. Unresolved stress can build up and create bigger anxiety in the long run.
4. **Difficulties in Work or Relationships**: Missing deadlines due to procrastination or substance use can cause conflicts or job trouble, which adds new layers of worry.

Recognizing Warning Signs

Sometimes it is obvious that a habit is harmful, but not always. Here are signs:

- You feel upset if you cannot do the habit (like if you run out of a favorite snack or cannot get online).
- You hide the habit from friends or family.
- You notice negative effects, like weight changes, financial issues, or conflicts with loved ones.
- You feel anxious without the habit, but calm down when you do it.
- You have tried to stop but keep going back.

If these sound familiar, it might be time to look at how to break the pattern.

Planning to Stop a Harmful Habit

1. **Identify the Habit Clearly**: It is best to name it specifically: "I have been drinking too much soda each day," or "I stay up until 3 a.m. scrolling on my phone."
2. **Discover the Trigger**: A trigger is the event or feeling that leads you to do the habit. Maybe you drink soda when stressed at work, or you play on your phone late because you cannot sleep. Knowing triggers helps you find ways to step in earlier.
3. **Set a Clear Goal**: Decide if you want to reduce the habit or remove it completely. For some, a full stop might be needed. For others, cutting down can be enough.
4. **Pick a Start Date**: Having a firm date or time to begin can boost your motivation.
5. **Line Up Support**: Tell a friend, join a group, or use an app to track progress. Accountability can keep you going when it is tough.

Replacing the Habit

Quitting a harmful habit is easier when you swap it with a healthier action. If you just remove the old habit without a new activity, you might feel a gap that leads to relapse. For example:

- **If You Overuse Screens**: Replace late-night phone use with reading a calm book or a short relaxation routine.
- **If You Smoke When Stressed**: Carry sugar-free gum or a small puzzle to distract you. Go for a quick walk instead of lighting a cigarette.
- **If You Snack on Sweets**: Keep chopped fruit or nuts on hand. When craving sugar, reach for these instead and pair them with a glass of water.
- **If You Procrastinate**: Use a simple timer method. Work for 20 minutes, then take a short break. This can give structure instead of last-minute panic.

The aim is not to rely purely on willpower but to build a new routine that offers similar relief without harming your health or fueling anxiety.

Handling Cravings or Urges

When trying to stop a habit, urges often appear:

1. **Pause and Breathe**: When an urge hits, do a quick breathing count—inhale for four seconds, hold one or two seconds, exhale for four. This can break the automatic move toward the habit.
2. **Delay Tactics**: Promise yourself you will wait 10 minutes before giving in. Often the urge might fade, or you find a healthier action to do instead.
3. **Distract**: Keep a list of short tasks or fun activities. As soon as you feel the craving, shift your focus to something else, like tidying a drawer or doing a simple puzzle.
4. **Visual Reminders**: A sticky note on your desk or a small charm you carry might remind you of your goal and why you are stopping the habit.

Dealing with Withdrawals

Some habits, like alcohol or certain drugs, can lead to real withdrawal signs when you quit. These might be headaches, trouble sleeping, or mood swings. If the habit is physically addictive, it can be risky to stop all at once without help. In that case:

- **Medical Input**: For serious substance issues, a health professional can guide you on safe ways to reduce use.
- **Hydration and Rest**: Drinking plenty of water, eating balanced meals, and resting can ease the body's stress.
- **Support System**: Let someone you trust know what you are going through. They can watch you for severe signs and offer moral help.
- **Gradual Cutting Down**: For some substances, lowering the dose step by step might be safer than going cold turkey.

Emotional Challenges

Even for non-addictive habits, stopping can stir up emotions:

- **Grief or Loss**: If the habit was a big part of your daily routine, letting it go might feel like losing a source of comfort.

- **Boredom**: You might find free time you used to spend on that habit, and not know what to do. Planning new, positive activities helps.
- **Anger or Irritability**: You might get annoyed at small things as your mind adjusts to living without the habit. This usually fades over time if you keep going.

Self-Talk for Breaking Habits

Encouraging self-talk helps you stay strong:

- **Positive Reminders**: "I can handle stress in healthier ways," or "This is tough, but I am getting stronger each day."
- **Avoid Self-Blame**: If you slip, do not call yourself names. Instead, say, "I had a setback, but I can learn from it and keep going."
- **Small Wins Count**: Each day or hour you avoid the habit is progress. Give yourself credit. This builds motivation to continue.

Avoiding High-Risk Moments

If you know certain times or places push you into the habit, plan ahead:

- **Social Triggers**: If friends invite you out for drinks but you want to cut back, suggest a different activity. If that is not possible, order a non-alcoholic drink.
- **Stress Points**: If you reach for a harmful habit after arguments or deadlines, create a small calming ritual instead, like a 5-minute stretch.
- **Environmental Changes**: Keep your home or workspace free of items linked to the habit. For example, if you are cutting out junk food, do not stock it. If you are trying to stop mindless phone use, keep the phone in another room.

Tracking Progress

Seeing your own improvement can strengthen your resolve:

- **Habit Tracker**: Use a chart or app to mark each day you avoid the habit.

- **Notice How You Feel**: After a while, check if you are sleeping better or if your mood is more stable.
- **Collect Encouragement**: Write down supportive words from friends or note changes in your anxiety levels. Reading them in tough times can help.

Handling Setbacks

It is common to slip up. One mistake does not erase all your progress. Think of it as a learning moment:

1. **Analyze the Slip**: Did it happen when you were tired, hungry, or stressed? Spot the cause.
2. **Plan a Fix**: Decide what you will do differently next time. For instance, if you gave in to late-night junk food because it was within reach, store it far away or do not buy it.
3. **Keep Going**: Do not let shame or guilt make you quit your goal. Recommit the next day. Each setback can shape a better plan.

When Professional Help Is Needed

Some habits are so rooted that outside help is necessary:

- **Support Groups**: Programs like Alcoholics Anonymous or other local groups can provide a sense of community and accountability.
- **Therapists**: A counselor can help address emotional issues behind the habit, teaching new coping skills.
- **Rehab or Treatment Centers**: For serious addictions, an inpatient or outpatient program might be the safest route.
- **Trusted Doctor**: If you suspect physical dependence, a doctor can guide you to resources for safely quitting.

Substitutes for Harmful Habits

It is not enough just to remove a habit. Filling that space with something better can keep you from returning to old patterns. Some ideas:

- **Exercise**: Even gentle routines like walking or beginner stretches can boost mood hormones.
- **Creative Projects**: Drawing, writing, or crafting can be a healthy outlet for stress.
- **Social Connections**: Instead of isolating, call a friend or join a club. Feeling connected lowers the urge to use quick-fix habits.
- **Nature Breaks**: Spending time outdoors has been linked to calmer moods. This can help you handle tension that once triggered the habit.
- **Mindful Breathing**: A few deep breaths can stand between you and the habit. Some people like to keep a small card in their wallet that reminds them of a short breathing sequence.

Breaking Negative Thought Loops

Thought habits can be just as harmful as physical ones. For example, constantly telling yourself "I'm useless" can ruin mood and keep you from taking healthy steps. Breaking negative loops needs:

1. **Spot the Thoughts**: Write them down when they arise. Notice if certain events trigger them.
2. **Question Them**: Ask if they are truly correct or if you are assuming the worst.
3. **Replace With Facts**: Think of times you handled things well, or consider a friend's viewpoint about your skills.
4. **Practice**: Each time a negative loop starts, interrupt it with a more balanced thought. This feels strange at first, but gets easier with repetition.

Rewards and Self-Care

While trying to stop a habit, a person might feel deprived. Building in small rewards can help:

- **Free Rewards**: Taking a relaxed bath, watching a funny clip, or reading an enjoyable book.
- **Low-Cost Rewards**: Buying a small item you have wanted after a week of success, like a new pen or a notebook for your thoughts.

- **Experience Rewards**: Plan a fun outing with a friend or try a new activity once you hit a milestone.

Giving yourself something positive can replace the old habit's short-term "feel-good" effect with a better, lasting sense of satisfaction.

Spotting Secret or Hidden Habits

Some harmful habits hide behind normal routines:

- **Overwork**: Working too many hours might look productive, but if it stops you from rest or personal time, it can raise anxiety.
- **People-Pleasing**: Always saying "yes" to requests, ignoring your own limits, can be a habit rooted in fear of letting others down.
- **Constant Negativity**: Quick to assume the worst in every situation, turning it into a reflex that increases stress.

Pay attention to daily life. If an action keeps fueling dread or drains your energy, it might be time to consider changes.

The Long-Term View

Quitting a habit is not just about the next few days. It is about creating a more stable life for the future. Once a habit is gone, you might feel more balanced energy or better self-esteem. Keep in mind:

- **Staying Alert**: The urge for the old habit can pop up again, even months later. Having a plan helps you handle sudden cravings.
- **Continued Learning**: As you remove one harmful habit, you might see others more clearly. Gradually fixing these can bring further mental relief.
- **Improved Relationships**: Stopping harmful habits often lets you connect better with loved ones, as you are more present and less stressed.

Hidden Effects of Stopping Harmful Habits

There can be surprising benefits:

1. **Better Sleep**: Without caffeine or late-night screen time, some people report easier sleep and more energy the next day.
2. **Clearer Thinking**: Less time spent on harmful habits can free the mind. You might handle tasks more smoothly or come up with creative ideas.
3. **Confidence Boost**: Doing something as difficult as quitting a harmful habit can make you feel more capable. This can carry over into handling other challenges.

Unique Tips for Stubborn Habits

1. **Change Routine Paths**: If you always buy sweets after work at the same shop, try a different route home so you are not tempted.
2. **Habit Bundling**: Pair a healthy activity you find boring with something you enjoy. For example, allow yourself to hear a favorite podcast only while walking or doing chores.
3. **Accountability Partner**: Find someone who checks in on you daily or weekly. Honesty helps you face your habit head-on.
4. **Tech Aids**: Use apps that block certain websites after a set amount of time, or that track your daily steps to encourage physical movement instead of sitting with the habit.

Combining Habit Change with Other Anxiety Work

Breaking harmful habits goes well with other anxiety methods like breathing exercises, balanced diets, or therapy. For example:

- **Therapy**: A therapist can help you see why you rely on a habit. Maybe it hides sadness or a fear from childhood. Understanding the root can make quitting easier.
- **Medication**: If anxiety is very strong, a doctor might suggest medication to help you get through the first phase of stopping a habit. Then you can use therapy or self-help steps to avoid slipping back.
- **Routine Building**: Filling your day with balanced tasks (like meal planning, short walks, or skill practice) can leave less empty space for the harmful habit to creep in.

Steps After Quitting

Once you stop or reduce a harmful habit, watch for:

- **New Confidence**: You might feel you can tackle other changes, like improving your diet or stepping up to a personal challenge.
- **Social Circles**: Friends who only joined you in the habit might fade out. Sometimes that is okay. You might look for new friends who support healthier living.
- **Dealing with Triggers**: You could still face triggers months later. Having a backup plan, like a text buddy or a relaxation drill, helps you handle these surprises.

Conclusion: Breaking Barriers

Harmful habits often arise because they fill a gap or give immediate relief from stress. But they keep you from finding long-term answers. By spotting these patterns, making a plan, and seeking help if needed, you can drop what weighs you down and open doors for healthier actions. This is a meaningful step in easing anxiety, because you remove extra sources of stress while also learning to handle worry in better ways.

In the next chapter, we will look at finding strength. Even when anxiety and harmful habits feel overwhelming, there are ways to see your own capabilities. Tapping into your inner resources can keep you motivated, especially when it feels like progress is slow. Understanding how to build a sense of inner power can make all the methods we have talked about even more effective. You might learn that you are stronger than you thought.

By breaking harmful habits, you clear obstacles that block real growth. Each day without those habits is a day you can focus on healthier patterns. Over time, the mental space that was taken by short-term fixes can be filled with lasting relief from anxiety and a sense of control over your life. This is not always easy, but with a steady approach, self-awareness, and the right support, big change is within reach.

CHAPTER 17: FINDING STRENGTH

Strength is not just about muscles or physical power. It is about having mental resources to handle challenges, stress, and change. When anxiety is present, it can make a person feel powerless or stuck. Learning to find strength within can help reduce those anxious feelings. This strength might show up in small daily actions or in the way you think about yourself. It can also be found in how you handle setbacks or unexpected events. In this chapter, we will look at why inner strength matters, how to discover it, and simple methods to make it grow. We will share tips that might not be common in regular guides, aiming to help you see that everyone has some form of strength, even if it feels hidden.

Why Inner Strength Matters

1. **Confidence in Tough Times**
   When anxiety rises, you might feel you have no control. Inner strength reminds you that you can face the moment. Even if the problem is big, strength can keep you from giving up right away.
2. **Reducing Fear of Failure**
   Fear of messing up can be paralyzing. Inner strength says, "I can try, and if I fail, I can learn something." This lessens the weight of worry.
3. **Greater Independence**
   If you rely only on others to calm your mind, you might feel helpless when they are not around. Building your own strength lets you handle many situations by yourself. It does not mean you refuse help; it means you have options.
4. **Better Recovery**
   Anxiety can sometimes knock you down for a bit. Inner strength helps you stand back up more quickly. Even if you feel nervous, you can still carry on with tasks or daily routines.

Understanding Strength Correctly

People often think of strength as being tough or never showing emotion. But real inner strength can include being honest about your feelings. If you are anxious, you do not have to hide it all the time. Instead, you acknowledge it and use coping skills. Real strength does not mean never feeling weak. It means choosing healthy ways to respond when worry or fear appears.

Also, strength is not one-size-fits-all. One person might show it by calmly facing conflict, another by asking for help when they need it, and another by being patient with themselves during slow progress. All these forms of strength are valid. Anxiety might tell you, "You are helpless," but that is often not true.

Sources of Inner Strength

1. **Past Challenges**
   Think back on times you handled difficulties—maybe an illness, a major exam, or a conflict at home. Even if it was messy, you came through it. That experience can remind you that you have the power to face problems again.
2. **Personal Values**
   Values are core beliefs that guide your actions, like honesty, kindness, or respect. Standing by these values can give you a stable sense of who you are, even when anxiety tries to sway you.
3. **Supportive Relationships**
   We all have moments of doubt. Having people who care—friends, family, or mentors—can help you see the strengths you miss. They might point out small wins that you overlooked.
4. **Faith or Philosophy**
   Some people draw strength from spiritual faith. Others find it in a personal philosophy, like believing in basic human goodness or the power of small efforts. Such frameworks can keep you going when you feel shaky.
5. **Skills and Interests**
   Doing something you are decent at—like cooking, organizing, or playing an instrument—can reveal a sense of capability. This capability can bleed over into other areas where you feel less confident.

Building Strength in Daily Life

1. **Small Victories**
   Aim for tasks slightly above your comfort level, but not so far they cause

extreme panic. Each time you succeed, write it down. Over time, you build a record of "I can do more than I thought."

2. **Routine Check-ins**
Spend a quiet minute each day asking, "What did I do well today?" and "What small skill did I use?" This helps you notice progress and encourages you to keep going.

3. **Physical Movement**
Light exercise can show you that your body can handle challenges. A short walk, gentle stretches, or simple exercises can build a sense of strength. Feeling your muscles work can remind you that you are not as fragile as anxiety might suggest.

4. **Help Others**
When you do something kind for someone else, it shows you have something to give. This can lift self-esteem. It might be giving advice, helping a neighbor carry groceries, or writing a supportive text to a friend. Such acts remind you that you have power to make a difference.

5. **Self-Aware Discipline**
Decide on a small discipline challenge—like waking up at a certain time, or tidying one area each day. Following through builds trust in yourself. It is not about perfection but about learning you can keep a promise to yourself.

Shifting Thoughts Toward Strength

1. **Notice Negative Labels**
Anxiety might label you as "weak" or "unable to handle anything." When you catch these labels in your mind, question them. Ask, "Is this a fair label, or am I ignoring times when I was strong?" Often, reality is more balanced.

2. **Replace with More Accurate Phrases**
For instance, if you think, "I am a failure," swap it for, "I have failed before, but I also have succeeded in some things." This does not pretend everything is great; it just keeps the view balanced.

3. **Use Gentle Encouragement**
Telling yourself, "I can handle this step," can be enough. You do not need to declare, "I will solve everything right now." Focus on the next small action.

4. **Check for Personal Evidence**
   Remind yourself of a time you solved a conflict, finished a tough task, or made it through a bad day. Such memories can push back against the lie that you cannot do anything.

Handling Doubt

Doubt can appear when trying to feel strong. You might think, "I am fooling myself," or "This is fake." Here are ways to handle doubt:

- **Accept It Exists**: Everyone has doubt. Do not fight it by yelling at yourself or trying to banish it instantly. Acknowledge it: "Yes, I feel unsure right now. That is normal."
- **Gather Facts**: If you are doubting your ability to manage a work project, list what steps you can take, or recall skills you have. Facts can help ease doubt's power.
- **Ask for Feedback**: A friend or colleague might see your strengths more clearly than you do. Hearing them say, "You handled that deadline last time, you can do it again," can remind you that your doubt is not the final truth.
- **Treat It Like a Signal**: Sometimes, doubt signals that you need more info or practice. If that is the case, use it as motivation to prepare or learn, rather than as proof that you are not capable.

Strength in Emotional Honesty

Being strong does not mean never admitting to anxiety or sadness. In fact, real strength can appear when you say, "I am anxious right now," while still taking sensible steps. Emotional honesty can reduce shame and help you find solutions:

1. **Label the Feeling**
   Saying, "I feel anxious," or "I feel tense," can stop the spiral of confusion. You have named it. Once named, you can respond better.
2. **Avoid Over-Apologizing**
   Some people say "I am sorry" for feeling anxious. But you do not need to apologize for your emotions. You can still be polite without blaming yourself for having feelings.

3. **Express in Healthy Ways**
   If you need to cry, do so in a safe place or with a supportive friend. If you need to release tension, some people find that writing, drawing, or talking to someone can help.
4. **Set Emotional Limits**
   While sharing can help, you do not have to spill every detail to everyone. Picking a safe person or a counselor can let you be honest without feeling exposed to negative reactions from those who might not understand.

Specific Exercises for Finding Strength

1. **Resilient Role Model**
   Think of someone you admire who overcame obstacles. It might be a historic figure, a family member, or a friend. Ask yourself how they might handle your current worry. This can give you ideas for strong actions.
2. **Mirror Encouragement**
   Though it might feel silly, look in the mirror and say one line about your power or a skill you have. For example, "I work hard, and I can tackle this problem." Even if it feels forced at first, repeating it can slowly build a more positive view.
3. **Fear-Setting**
   Write down your fear in detail, including worst outcomes. Then list what steps you could take if the worst happened. Often, you see that even in a bad situation, you would still have options. This knowledge can lessen anxiety and show you that you are more prepared than you thought.
4. **Quiet Body Check**
   When anxiety spikes, pause and check your body from toes to head. Notice tension, then try to release it. As you feel your muscles relax, it reminds you that you can influence how your body feels. This small moment of control can hint at deeper strength.

Changing How You View Setbacks

Everyone faces setbacks, and anxiety might scream that a setback is final. But a strong approach sees setbacks as part of life. To handle them:

- **Identify What Went Wrong**: Maybe you missed a deadline or had a panic attack during a speech. Write down what actually happened, avoiding harsh judgment.
- **Find Lessons**: Did you skip some steps? Were you overly tired? Did you ignore early signs of stress? Use this info to adjust next time.
- **Stay Kind to Yourself**: A slip does not erase all your progress. It just shows you what still needs work. Inner strength grows from trying again.

Over time, this method can reframe setbacks from "proof of weakness" to "chances to learn."

The Link Between Strength and Hope

Hope is the belief that things can improve or that you can find a way forward. Strength feeds on hope, and hope can grow from seeing signs of strength. If you have even a small sign that you can face difficulties—like finishing a task under stress—this can spark hope. Then, hope helps you attempt the next challenge, which builds more strength. They support each other. Anxiety can weaken hope, but if you keep track of any sign of progress, you can fuel hope again.

Finding Strength with Others

Strength is not always a solo activity. Sometimes, real strength involves reaching out:

- **Group or Community**: Joining a supportive group can remind you that you are not alone. It takes courage to show up and share your story. That is strength.
- **Shared Efforts**: If you and a friend both have goals (like dealing with social anxiety or finishing a project at work), you can keep each other accountable. This mutual support can boost confidence.
- **Mentoring**: If you are further along in handling a certain fear or skill, you might mentor someone else. Teaching or guiding another person can show you how much you have learned, revealing hidden strengths.

Balancing Strength and Rest

It is easy to confuse strength with constant effort. But everyone needs rest. Pushing yourself endlessly can lead to burnout and even higher anxiety. True strength recognizes the value of breaks:

1. **Allow Relaxation**: Taking breaks, having fun, or enjoying quiet moments does not mean you are lazy. It recharges your mental energy.
2. **Respect Your Limits**: If you feel extremely tired or you have a headache, forcing yourself to keep going might do more harm. Strength can mean wisely taking a pause.
3. **Vary Your Activities**: If you are working on a tough project, switch occasionally to simpler tasks. This shift in focus can keep you from mental fatigue.

When you plan rest, you are preserving your energy to face challenges more effectively. A well-rested mind handles anxiety better than one that is drained.

Navigating Criticism or Negativity

Others might judge you or belittle your efforts. Anxiety might increase if you feel attacked or misunderstood. Using your inner strength in these moments can look like:

- **Staying Calm**: Instead of reacting with anger, take a breath, and decide if you should respond. Sometimes a simple, calm reply is better than a heated defense.
- **Knowing Your Worth**: If you have built a sense of your values and skills, random negative comments might hurt less. You can think, "They do not see the full picture of who I am."
- **Choosing Battles**: Not every comment needs a debate. Sometimes you can walk away, or politely end the discussion. Strength can be not fighting every negative remark.

Looking for Strength Outside Yourself

While inner strength is key, reminders in the outside world can help:

1. **Daily Affirmations Around You**
   Place short, strong lines on sticky notes in places you see often, like a desk or a bathroom mirror. Reading them keeps you connected to a positive mindset.
2. **Symbols or Items**
   Some people wear a bracelet or keep a small object in their pocket that reminds them of their goals. When anxiety flares up, touching the item can bring comfort.
3. **Reading or Listening**
   Some books, songs, or podcasts have messages of resilience. Dipping into them can refresh your sense of strength. Just be mindful of not overloading on content that might raise stress.

Uncommon Ways to Boost Strength

1. **Learn Something New**
   Trying a new skill—like a simple language lesson or a craft—lets you see you can grow. Each time you grasp a new word or create a small project, you prove you can change.
2. **Mental "Strength" Workouts**
   Just as people do physical workouts, you can do mental ones. For example, pick a mild stressor on purpose, like completing a puzzle with a time limit. Practice staying calm through it. Over time, you build mental stamina.
3. **Make a "Can Do" List**
   People often have to-do lists that feel heavy. Instead, make a "can do" list: write down tasks or things you already handle well. This reminds you that you are not starting from zero.
4. **Challenge the Unknown**
   Sometimes, anxiety feeds on the unknown. If there is a safe but unfamiliar thing you can try—a new route home, a different grocery store, or a simple event—trying it builds the idea that you can face newness without falling apart.

Using Strength to Reduce Anxiety Patterns

As you grow in strength, you can apply it to anxiety patterns you have spotted. For instance, if your pattern is to avoid certain social events, use your newfound confidence to attend one small gathering. If your pattern is negative thinking at night, use your self-belief to correct those thoughts when they appear. Over time, your personal power can unlearn long-held fear responses.

Staying Motivated When Progress Is Slow

Progress with anxiety is not always quick. You might see improvements and then feel stuck:

- **Remember Why You Started**: Recall the pain of anxiety controlling your life. This can keep you going.
- **Check How Far You Have Come**: Looking back at an old journal entry or talking with a friend about your early struggles can reveal that you have grown, even if it feels slow.
- **Try New Angles**: If you feel truly stuck, consider a different strategy. Maybe a new relaxation exercise, a different kind of therapy, or seeking advice from a mentor.

Accepting That Strength Fluctuates

You might have times where you feel very strong and times where you feel less so. This is normal. Body energy, outside stress, and many other factors can influence your sense of power on any given day. Recognizing that there will be ups and downs helps you avoid panic when a strong day is followed by a weaker one. You can think, "I had a rough moment, but I can rise again, as I have before."

Putting It All Together

Finding strength is about noticing what you can do, what you can handle, and what you can learn. It involves small actions each day that slowly change the way you see yourself and your ability to face anxiety. It also means being honest about your feelings, forgiving yourself for mistakes, and knowing that you can keep trying. There is no magic switch that turns you instantly into a fearless person. Instead, it is a step-by-step path of understanding your capacity, training your mind to spot opportunities instead of dead ends, and gathering facts that show you are more capable than you once believed.

When anxiety tries to whisper that you are weak or that you should quit, you can remember moments when you showed even a bit of courage. Inner strength does not announce itself with big fanfare. It grows quietly, in repeated attempts and simple daily wins. Over time, it becomes something you trust more than the old fearful voices.

In the next chapter, we will look at dealing with uncertainty. Anxiety often grows when the future is unclear or when we do not know what will happen next. Building on the idea of inner strength, we will see how acceptance of the unknown, practical planning, and a balanced mindset can help you stay calm even when life does not give clear answers. By pairing the growth of personal power with these approaches to uncertainty, you can continue to lower anxiety and live with more steadiness.

CHAPTER 18: DEALING WITH UNCERTAINTY

Uncertainty is a large source of anxiety. When people do not know what is coming, they can feel tense, worried, or on edge. It might be uncertainty about health, finances, relationships, or world events. Everyone faces unknown outcomes, but those with anxiety might find the lack of control extra upsetting. Yet, uncertainty is part of life. Learning to live with it, plan around it, and see it in a calmer way can reduce a lot of stress. This chapter will explore why the unknown feels so scary, how to handle it, and specific steps to stay balanced when events are not clear.

Why Uncertainty Triggers Anxiety

1. **Desire for Control**
   People often feel safer when they can predict the next steps. Anxiety flares up when the path ahead looks murky. The brain may try to guess the worst outcome as a way to prepare, but this can lead to constant worry.
2. **Fear of Negative Surprises**
   Uncertainty can bring up thoughts like, "What if something bad happens that I did not plan for?" or "What if I cannot handle it?" This type of thinking can keep the mind stuck in a loop of possible disasters.
3. **Past Experiences**
   A rough event in the past, like an unexpected job loss or sudden illness, can make the person extra alert. They might think, "I did not see it coming last time, so now I must always watch out."
4. **Comparison to Others**
   Seeing friends or coworkers who seem to have "everything figured out" can heighten anxiety. The person might believe everyone else knows exactly what is next, even though many people face doubts silently.

Shifting How You View Uncertainty

Instead of treating uncertainty as an enemy, you can try a different perspective:

1. **Accept It as Normal**
   Life is full of things we cannot fully predict. Even the weather can shift quickly. Recognizing that some unknowns are natural helps you stop seeing them as personal threats.
2. **Focus on What You Can Influence**
   While you cannot control everything, there are usually small steps or choices you can make. Shifting your focus to these can lower the sense of helplessness.
3. **Expect Some Surprises**
   If you go into a situation expecting that surprises might come up, then each surprise feels less like a shock. You might say, "I will do what I can, and if something unexpected happens, I will handle it."
4. **Remember Past Adjustments**
   Think about how you handled unknown events before. Perhaps you found a new job after layoffs or solved a sudden home repair issue. Those memories show that even if you did not see something coming, you coped in some way.

Tools for Living with the Unknown

1. **Practical Planning**
   Make general plans for likely scenarios. For example, if you worry about job security, you could update your resume or put some money aside if possible. This does not mean you obsess over every detail, but it can reduce panic if something happens.
2. **Limit Hypotheticals**
   The mind might spin out many "what if" thoughts. You can set a boundary, like "I will consider one or two likely scenarios, then stop and move on." Constantly listing dozens of possible outcomes can raise anxiety rather than help.
3. **Problem-Solving Steps**
   If there is a real risk, use a systematic approach:
   - Define the concern clearly.
   - Brainstorm ways to handle it.
   - Pick the most workable plan.
   - Remind yourself you have at least a partial strategy.
4. **Mindful Distraction**
   After you have done what you reasonably can, find a healthy distraction,

such as a hobby or calling a friend. Overthinking does not remove uncertainty; it often just makes you more anxious.

Reducing Overthinking

Overthinking is trying to solve or perfect every detail in your head, which can drain mental energy. Some ways to cut back on it:

- **Set "Worry Time"**: Assign a short block of time each day to think about your worries. If a worry pops up outside that time, you can tell yourself, "I will look at that in my worry time."
- **Postpone Repetitive Thoughts**: If you catch yourself circling back to the same question, gently say "stop" to yourself and switch tasks.
- **Stay in the Present**: Focus on immediate senses or tasks. If you are washing dishes, notice the water temperature, the sound, or how the dish feels in your hand. This lowers the mind's swirl of future-based worry.

Handling Big "What Ifs"

1. **List Realistic Probabilities**
   Anxiety might paint everything as a 90% chance of doom, but the actual probability might be far lower. Doing a realistic check can help. For instance, if you fear a plane crash but know it is statistically rare, that fact can reduce panic.
2. **Ask, "Can I Cope if This Happens?"**
   Usually, the answer is "yes, though it would be hard." Knowing you could cope if the worst happened (by seeking help, changing plans, etc.) can make uncertainty less overwhelming.
3. **Avoid Gathering Endless Data**
   Sometimes, you look up a lot of info online, hoping to become sure about everything. But too much info can contradict itself, causing more confusion. There is a balance between being informed and being overloaded.
4. **Take a Single Next Step**
   If you are anxious about a possible illness, perhaps the next step is booking a checkup or following basic health guidelines. Doing that step can calm the sense of panic about the unknown.

The Role of Flexibility

Flexibility is the ability to adjust when things do not go as planned. This trait helps with uncertainty because you are not locked into one rigid outcome:

- **Practice Plan B Thinking**
  If Plan A fails, what is Plan B? This is not about expecting failure but acknowledging multiple paths to success.
- **Stay Open to Learning**
  When something unexpected happens, ask, "What can I learn here?" This can turn a scary unknown into a lesson or an opportunity.
- **Self-Trust in Adaptation**
  Remind yourself that you can adapt, even if it is uncomfortable. Each time you do so, you gain more evidence that you handle the unknown better than you thought.

Accepting Partial Answers

Sometimes, you get partial clues about the future but not the full picture. Anxiety might push you to gather more details, but life may not offer them yet. In these cases:

1. **Use the Info You Do Have**
   Work with whatever facts are available. If it is incomplete, do the best you can.
2. **Set a Review Date**
   If the situation might change later, mark a date on the calendar to check for updates. This prevents you from obsessively checking every hour.
3. **Stay Engaged Elsewhere**
   Keep living your life in other areas. Focusing on relationships, hobbies, or personal growth can keep the unknown from dominating every moment.

Healthy Ways to Cope with Anxiety from Uncertainty

1. **Breathing Drills**
   Use a simple pattern: inhale for four, hold for two, exhale for four. This can calm physical tension.

2. **Grounding Exercises**
   Name five objects you see, four things you can touch, three sounds you hear, two smells you notice, and one taste or sense in your mouth. This focuses your mind on the present reality instead of future panic.
3. **Exercise or Movement**
   A short walk or some stretches can help release stress hormones. Even pacing around the room can break the cycle of anxious thinking.
4. **Creative Outlets**
   Writing, painting, or playing music lets you express worry in a constructive way. Instead of spiraling in your head, you put the energy into creating something.

Staying Balanced in an Unpredictable World

The world is full of sudden changes, like economic shifts, natural events, or health concerns. To stay balanced:

- **Check News in Moderation**
  Constantly reading updates can fuel panic. Pick trusted sources, check them briefly, then step away.
- **Gather Practical Tools**
  Keep basic supplies at home, have emergency contacts, and know local safety guidelines. Feeling prepared can reduce fear.
- **Find Common Ground**
  Talking with others about how they cope can help you feel less alone. Many people share similar worries, and trading tips can build group resilience.

Strengthening Mental Habits for Uncertain Times

1. **Seek Support**
   If you have a close friend or a counselor, discuss your fears about the unknown. Sometimes hearing an outside view helps you see that you have done enough.
2. **Avoid Perfectionism**
   Uncertainty often means you cannot do everything flawlessly. Trying to be perfect in the face of the unknown can increase frustration.

3. **Practice Letting Go**
   If you have done your part—like applying for a job or studying for a test—there might be a waiting period. Learning to let go of the rest can free up mental space for other things.

Replacing Catastrophic Thoughts

Anxiety likes to paint the worst possible future, a process called catastrophic thinking. To fight this pattern:

- **Identify the Catastrophe**
  Notice statements like, "If this event goes wrong, my entire life is ruined."
- **Use Evidence**
  Challenge it with real facts: "I have had bad events before, but my entire life was not ruined. I found ways to cope or adapt."
- **Scale It Down**
  If you catch yourself using extreme words like "always," "never," or "ruin," try softer words like "sometimes," "maybe," or "difficult."
- **Place It in a Timeline**
  Ask, "Will this still matter to me in a month or a year?" Often, the answer is smaller than your initial fear suggests.

Finding Growth in Uncertainty

Though it might sound odd, some people find that uncertainty forces them to explore new paths or build new strengths. For example, if a job is lost unexpectedly, you might discover a new line of work or skill you never considered. If a planned trip is canceled, you might find a different local activity that turns out to be special. Being open to unexpected doors can lessen anxiety's hold on you.

Personal Practices to Handle the Unknown

1. **Daily Reminder**
   Write or say a short phrase like, "I can manage what I can and let the rest be," each morning.

2. **Regular Self-Check**
   Ask yourself: "What uncertainty is on my mind today, and have I done what I reasonably can about it?" If yes, release the rest until more info comes.
3. **Align Actions with Values**
   Rather than chasing total security, aim to live by your values each day. This might mean being kind, creative, or honest, regardless of uncertain outcomes.

How to Plan Without Obsessing

Planning is healthy when it helps you stay organized. It becomes obsessive when you cannot stop planning multiple worst-case scenarios. To avoid over-planning:

- **Set a Time Limit**
  Decide how long you will spend planning. When that time is up, move to another task.
- **Pick the Priority**
  Sort possible issues by how likely or important they are. Tackle the top one or two. Let the minor ones go if they are not urgent.
- **Involve Others**
  If you are stuck, ask a friend or family member to review your plan. They might see that you are overdoing it or missing a simpler path.

Keeping Hope Alive

Uncertainty can make the future look dark. But there are ways to keep hope:

1. **Focus on Small Good Things**
   Even if tomorrow is unclear, you can notice a kind act someone did, or a nice event that happened. This balances out fear.
2. **Recall Past Success**
   If you made it through uncertain times before—like finishing a tough school program or navigating a move—this shows you can face unknowns again.
3. **Connect with Others Who Share Optimism**
   Spend time with people who look for solutions rather than dwelling on doom. Their attitude can rub off on you.

When to Seek Extra Help

Sometimes, the stress of uncertainty becomes too big to handle alone:

- **Anxiety Is Constant**
  If you cannot sleep or concentrate, or your worry stops you from doing normal tasks, it might be time for professional input.
- **Physical Symptoms**
  Constant headaches, stomach trouble, or rapid heartbeat could be signs that anxiety is wearing you down. A doctor can help you rule out other causes and suggest ways to cope.
- **Negative Coping**
  If you find yourself turning to harmful habits (like substance use) more frequently because you cannot deal with the unknown, seeking help can stop the cycle.

Therapy, counseling, or support groups can teach you advanced ways to handle the fear of uncertainty. They might use techniques like exposure to small risks, or structured thinking exercises, to help you become more relaxed with not knowing all the answers.

Dealing with Global or Large-Scale Unknowns

Events like economic shifts or health crises can feel overwhelming because you, as an individual, cannot fix them alone. Strategies include:

- **Focus on Local Influence**
  See what actions you can take in your community or personal circle, such as small safety steps or offering help to neighbors.
- **Limit Negative Input**
  Endless doom-filled news can raise panic. Keep up to date but avoid checking news non-stop.
- **Gather Support**
  Talk with friends or join local groups that share practical tips or emotional help during large-scale events.

Bringing It All Together

Uncertainty does not need to ruin your peace. By accepting that some unknowns are natural, focusing on what you can do, limiting endless "what if" thinking, and practicing self-care, you reduce the grip anxiety has on you. It can help to see yourself as flexible, resourceful, and able to handle surprises. When new questions pop up, you can think, "I do not have all the answers right now, but I can manage what is in front of me and adapt as needed."

Life rarely gives us total certainty. Even so, learning to live with partial information while keeping a balanced mind can free up energy. You can spend less time worrying about the future and more time engaging with the present. This does not mean ignoring real concerns. It means addressing them as effectively as you can, then stepping away from pointless fear.

In the next chapters, we will cover giving and receiving support, then we will move on to maintaining progress over the long run. These topics continue to build on everything we have discussed so far. Anxiety management is not just about stopping nervous thoughts. It is also about staying connected with others, having healthy relationships, and setting a stable path for the future. By dealing calmly with uncertainty now, you create the groundwork for strong connections and steady personal growth later on.

CHAPTER 19: GIVING AND RECEIVING SUPPORT

Getting support from others and giving support to others can help reduce anxiety. It also strengthens connections. Many people feel anxious alone, but sharing worries or lending an ear can offer relief. Yet asking for help is not always easy. Some worry they will be a burden. Others do not know how to give support in a helpful way. This chapter explains the basics of giving and receiving support. It also looks at some less-common ideas about how support works, so you can use it in your daily life.

Why Support Matters

1. **Shared Burden**
   Anxiety often grows when a person carries all their stress alone. Talking about it can lighten that load. Sometimes, just saying words out loud relieves tension, even before solutions appear.
2. **Fresh Perspective**
   A friend or relative can see a problem from another angle. They might notice a simple fix you have overlooked. They might remind you of strengths you forgot you had.
3. **Feeling Understood**
   Anxiety can trick you into thinking you are strange or alone in your fears. Realizing someone else hears you, or even shares similar worries, can reduce shame and lower stress.
4. **Improved Mood**
   Positive social contact can boost mood. Research suggests that being around caring individuals helps the body produce feel-good chemicals. It does not remove all anxiety, but it can provide calmness.

Barriers to Asking for Help

1. **Fear of Judgment**
   A person might worry that friends will think less of them for having anxiety. They might think, "People will see me as weak if I speak up."
2. **Concern About Burdening Others**
   They might think, "I do not want to add to someone else's problems." This can stop them from seeking help, even when they need it.

3. **Belief That They Should Cope Alone**
   In some cultures or families, there is an idea that handling anxiety alone is a sign of strength. Asking for help might feel like failure. However, learning to accept help can be a healthy choice.
4. **Not Knowing Where to Start**
   Some people genuinely do not know who or how to ask. They might not have a close circle. They might not be sure if a professional is necessary or if friends are enough.

Overcoming the Hesitation

1. **Start with a Trustworthy Person**
   Pick someone you trust at a basic level, like a kind friend, sibling, or counselor at school. You do not have to reveal everything at once—just try to open a conversation about feeling stressed or uneasy.
2. **Use Simple Statements**
   You can say, "I have been feeling really worried," or "Sometimes I get very anxious, and it's hard to handle." You do not need perfect words. Honesty and clarity can be enough.
3. **Seek Common Experiences**
   Sometimes, it helps to join a small group or an online forum about anxiety or stress. Seeing others discuss the same feelings can lower your fear of judgment.
4. **Practice Asking for Specific Help**
   Instead of, "I need help," you could say, "Could we talk for a few minutes? I have been overwhelmed lately," or "Would you mind if I text you when I feel panic coming on?" Such direct requests can help others know how to respond.

The Art of Giving Support

1. **Listen More Than You Talk**
   When a friend or family member shares anxious thoughts, you might want to fix everything right away. But often, they need someone to listen. Let them finish talking before you offer any advice. Reflect back what they

said, like "So you're feeling scared about your job—did I get that right?" This shows you heard them correctly.

2. **Use Empathy**
Empathy means trying to understand how someone feels, even if you are not in the exact situation. Phrases like, "That sounds really tough," or "I can see why that's stressing you," show respect for their feelings.

3. **Offer Help Without Demanding**
If you have a suggestion, ask if the person wants it. You might say, "I have an idea—would you like to hear it?" Some people may only want to vent. Others may be happy to get input.

4. **Avoid Minimizing**
Saying, "It's not a big deal," or "Other people have worse problems," can make someone feel unheard. Every person's anxiety is real to them, and comparing does not usually help.

5. **Check In Later**
If you talk with someone today, you might send a short text tomorrow: "How are you feeling now?" This shows ongoing care, not just a one-time event.

Practical Support vs. Emotional Support

1. **Practical Support**
This involves taking some actions or tasks off someone's plate. For example, cooking a meal for a friend who is overwhelmed, or helping them study if they worry about an exam. It can reduce immediate stress.

2. **Emotional Support**
This involves listening, encouraging, and reassuring. It does not solve the practical problem, but it helps the person feel safer and less alone.

Some people need both. For instance, a person who is anxious about messy finances might need emotional support while also receiving practical help—like going through bills together. Asking which type of support the person wants can avoid confusion.

Setting Boundaries When Helping

1. **Respect Your Limits**
   You cannot carry someone else's anxiety all the time. If providing support becomes too heavy or constant, it may harm your own mental health. It is okay to say, "I want to help, but I also need breaks sometimes."
2. **Suggest Other Resources**
   If you feel you are not equipped to handle intense anxiety or deeper issues, you can gently suggest they see a professional, like a counselor or doctor. You could say, "I care about you a lot, and I think a professional might offer more help than I can."
3. **Avoid Taking Control**
   If a friend is anxious, it can be tempting to solve everything for them. But they need the chance to grow their own coping skills. Offer ideas or help, but do not run their life.
4. **Communicate Clearly**
   If you can only chat in the evenings due to work, tell the person. If you feel tired and cannot talk about anxious topics tonight, say so kindly. Clear communication prevents misunderstandings.

Group Support and Community

1. **Peer Support Groups**
   Some people benefit from groups where each member faces anxiety or stress. They share stories, tips, and moral support. It is a space to feel normal about struggles.
2. **Faith or Community Centers**
   Some places of worship or community centers hold gatherings where people support each other emotionally. If that aligns with your background, it might be a helpful resource.
3. **Online Forums**
   In today's world, the internet offers many discussion boards and social groups. Carefully choose places that feel positive and supportive, rather than negative or harsh.
4. **Making New Contacts**
   If you do not have close friends, you can expand your circle by joining clubs, volunteer groups, or classes. Building new connections might take time, but each contact can be a step forward.

Support from Professionals

1. **Therapists and Counselors**
    They have training to listen, guide, and teach coping tools. Talking to a professional can bring faster results than struggling alone. They can help you see patterns, rework negative thoughts, or handle panic spells.
2. **Support Hotlines**
    If anxiety peaks suddenly, a hotline can be a place to talk without committing to long-term therapy. Volunteers are trained to respond with calmness and empathy.
3. **EAP (Employee Assistance Program)**
    Some workplaces have these programs, offering short-term counseling or referrals for employees. If stress is linked to work, this might be a good route.
4. **School Counselors**
    Students often have free access to a school counselor or mental health professional. They can help with academic worries, social fears, or personal issues. It is a real resource many do not use.

Being a Good Support Receiver

1. **Express Thanks**
    If a friend or counselor spends time listening to you, a simple thank you can encourage them. It also reminds you not to take support for granted.
2. **Return the Favor (If Possible)**
    Support is not always one-way. Even if you feel anxious, you can still ask about your friend's life or lend an ear. Helping someone else might also shift your mind off your own worries.
3. **Honor Agreements**
    If a friend sets a boundary, respect it. For example, if they say they are unavailable after 9 p.m., try not to call them at midnight with a crisis unless it is truly an emergency.
4. **Be Honest About Progress**
    If you are following a friend's suggestion, let them know what worked or what did not. This feedback can help them understand your situation better.

Avoiding Toxic Support Dynamics

1. **Guilt-Tripping**
   Sometimes, a person tries to gain help by making others feel guilty. This can harm the relationship. It is better to be direct about needs rather than using guilt.
2. **Drama Cycles**
   Some individuals jump from crisis to crisis, always expecting everyone to drop everything. If you notice this pattern, step back and consider if it is real anxiety or a habit of seeking attention.
3. **Over-Reliance**
   Relying on one single friend for all emotional support can be risky. If that friend gets busy or needs time off, you might feel abandoned. Building a support network of multiple people or resources is healthier.
4. **Hiding Major Concerns**
   If you only share mild worries but hide bigger issues, no one can help with the root problem. Practice opening up a bit more if you want meaningful support.

Giving Support to Yourself

1. **Self-Compassion**
   Speak to yourself in a friendly tone, the way you would talk to someone you care about. If you make a mistake, try, "I messed up, but I will learn from this," rather than harsh self-criticism.
2. **Rewarding Tiny Steps**
   If you face a fear, even if the outcome is not perfect, praise yourself: "I tried. That's progress." Over time, these small praises add up.
3. **Set Up Comfort Habits**
   This might be sipping a warm drink when anxious, or a quick break to breathe. A small routine that grounds you can be a form of self-support.
4. **Know Your Patterns**
   If you see that late-night overthinking often sparks panic, plan ahead for that time. You might read a calming book or do simple stretches before bed. This preempts the anxiety cycle.

Support in Different Life Settings

1. **Family Setting**
   Some families are warm and open, while others can be critical. If your family is supportive, share your worries. If they are not, seek support elsewhere. You can still love your family but choose to confide in a friend or professional who respects your feelings.
2. **Work Setting**
   Telling a boss or coworker about your anxiety can be tricky. Sometimes, a quick mention like, "I'm dealing with stress right now," might be enough to explain a drop in your usual performance. But you do not have to reveal everything if you fear stigma. A mental health day or an EAP can be good alternatives.
3. **School Setting**
   Students might get anxious about grades or social acceptance. A supportive teacher or school counselor can be a big help. Classmates might also bond over shared worries, forming study groups or chat sessions.
4. **Online or Remote**
   If you live far from close friends, video calls or messaging apps can keep you connected. Virtual support groups also exist. Be cautious about privacy and choose reliable forums if you share personal details.

Respecting Differences in Giving and Receiving

Each person has a unique style of handling anxiety. One friend might want to talk for hours, another might prefer short texts. One person might like direct advice, another might just want quiet listening. It helps to ask, "How would you like me to support you?" or "Do you want my thoughts, or do you just want someone to listen?" This clarity prevents conflicts.

When Support Is Not Enough

Even the best friend or group might not be able to fully handle severe anxiety. If you notice serious signs:

- Panic attacks that happen often.
- Ongoing thoughts of self-harm or harming others.
- Inability to do basic activities like going to work or maintaining hygiene.
- Severe substance misuse.

In these cases, professional help is strongly advised. Telling someone, "You might benefit from seeing a doctor or counselor," is an act of care, not an insult.

Creative Approaches

1. **Support Journals**
   You and a friend can exchange short letters in a shared journal. Each can write updates or encouraging words. This can be a slower-paced way to connect if phone calls are hard.
2. **Buddy Challenges**
   If you both want to handle anxiety better, try a friendly challenge: each day, do one small action that fights avoidance or negativity, then share your results. This mutual accountability can be motivating.
3. **Collaborative Problem-Solving**
   If you both have a similar worry, talk about it and make a plan together. For example, if both fear public speaking, you could practice mini-presentations for each other in private.
4. **Multi-Person Support**
   Sometimes, a group of three or four people can meet regularly (in person or online) to discuss goals, stress, or progress. Having multiple viewpoints can spark more ideas.

Building a Culture of Support

If you want to encourage supportive attitudes:

- **Model Openness**: Let people see you handle stress in a balanced way and occasionally ask for help. This can give them permission to do the same.
- **Share Resources**: If you find a good article or technique, mention it casually. "I read about a breathing trick that helps reduce worry—want to hear about it?"
- **Celebrate Small Gains**: When someone you know does something brave, you can say, "That's great progress. I'm proud of you," or simply, "You did

well." This can reinforce a supportive environment without using flashy language.
- **Stay Aware of Boundaries**: Being supportive does not mean you must fix every problem or become everyone's helper 24/7. Encourage others to learn self-help skills as well.

Handling Disagreements in Support

Sometimes, you try to help but conflict arises. Maybe the person feels pushed, or you sense they are ignoring your efforts. Calm communication can solve many of these issues:

- **Clarify Intent**: "I care, and I wanted to see if you were open to hearing an idea. I don't want to force anything on you."
- **Respect "No"**: If they do not want to try your suggestion, step back. People need to own their choices.
- **Express Feelings Kindly**: If you feel unappreciated, you could say, "I want to help, but I feel my efforts are not noticed. Can we talk about how I can help in a way that you would find useful?"
- **Consider Timing**: Right when someone is in deep panic might not be the best moment to push solutions. Wait until they calm down, then bring up ideas.

Monitoring Support Over Time

Over the months and years, the nature of support might change. A friend who once talked to you daily might get busier. You might move or switch workplaces. People's own issues can also change. Keep the following in mind:

- **Periodically Check In**: Ask, "Are we still helping each other in the best way, or do we need a new approach?"
- **Adapt**: If a friend no longer has time for daily messages, maybe weekly calls or a monthly meet-up works better.
- **Stay Open to New Connections**: Life changes bring new people. Being willing to accept new support can keep you from feeling alone if older connections drift away.

Putting Support into Action

1. **Create a Short Contact List**
   List two or three people you trust to talk with if anxiety spikes. Also list any hotline or professional resource that you might call.
2. **Plan a Support Chat**
   If you have not opened up to someone yet, pick a day or time to do so. It might be a quick text or a coffee invite. Just mention you have something on your mind.
3. **Offer a Hand**
   If you know a friend is anxious about a test or a presentation, you might say, "Would it help to practice once with me?" or "Need a quick call to talk things over?"
4. **Be Proactive**
   Sometimes, you see that a friend is anxious but not saying it. A gentle "How are you doing lately?" can let them know you are there. They might open up if they feel safe.

Looking Ahead

Giving and receiving support is part of a healthy life, especially when facing anxiety. No one has to handle worry all by themselves. By learning to share concerns and encourage each other, you can lower stress levels and create stronger bonds. This chapter explored why support is important, how to get and give it, and ways to keep boundaries healthy.

The next (and final) chapter will focus on maintaining progress over time. Anxiety management is not just a one-time event. After learning so many methods—routines, thinking strategies, ways to find strength, and using social support—how do you keep these gains? The final chapter will look at ways to prevent setbacks, adjust to new challenges, and keep up the calm mindset you have built. The aim is to keep moving forward, using everything you have learned, so that worry does not take over again. By mastering the art of support and combining it with healthy habits, you set the stage for a life that is more steady, even when stress appears.

CHAPTER 20: MAINTAINING PROGRESS

You have learned a great deal about anxiety, how it works, how to reduce it, and how to build supportive habits. The big question now is how to keep these gains for the long haul. Anxiety can come in waves. Even if it eases for a while, stress can return with changes in work, health, family, or other areas. Maintaining progress is about treating mental well-being like a garden—something you water and check on regularly so it does not wither. In this final chapter, we will explore ways to stay on track, adapt to future stress, and live a life that is not dominated by worry. We will also share small but powerful tips you can use to stay motivated and balanced.

Why Maintenance Is Important

1. **Prevent Relapse**
   If you stop the healthy practices that helped you manage anxiety, old patterns may reappear. Regular use of coping skills can protect against a return of high worry.
2. **Handle New Challenges**
   Life changes—getting a new job, moving to a different city, facing health issues—can stir fresh anxiety. A solid maintenance plan means you have the tools ready to adjust.
3. **Build on Growth**
   Maintaining progress is not just about avoiding setbacks. It can also mean continuing to grow, taking on new goals, and finding more satisfaction in everyday life.
4. **Boost Self-Trust**
   Sticking with healthy habits over time shows you can depend on yourself, which builds confidence. Each small success in following your plan is proof that you can keep anxiety in check.

Key Components of a Maintenance Plan

1. **Regular Check-Ins**
   At least once a week, pause and ask: "How am I feeling? Has worry started

creeping back? Am I still using the methods I learned?" This small habit helps you catch early signs of trouble.

2. **Updated Routines**
If your schedule changes—like switching jobs or taking on new responsibilities—adjust your routines. For example, if you used to do a morning breathing exercise but now must leave the house earlier, you might do a shorter version or switch to a midday break.

3. **Support System**
Keep in touch with supportive friends, counselors, or groups. Even if you feel better, an ongoing connection can be a safety net. You never know when you might need a listening ear again.

4. **Physical Health**
Sleep, nutrition, and gentle exercise remain major factors in mental well-being. If you slip in these areas, anxiety can rise. Scheduling them as priorities can maintain your gains.

Early Warning Signs of Slipping

1. **Avoidance Returns**
If you start avoiding tasks or social events again, it might mean worry is growing. Noticing this quickly can prompt you to reapply your coping strategies.

2. **Racing Negative Thoughts**
Do you find your mind jumping back to worst-case scenarios more often? This can be a sign that you should refresh your thought-checking tools.

3. **Change in Mood or Energy**
Feeling more irritable, tired, or restless could mean anxiety is creeping back. Comparing how you felt in calmer times can help you notice the shift.

4. **Lack of Motivation**
If you stop caring about the habits or routines that used to help you—like daily walks or journaling—that can signal a slip in progress. Motivation might drop when you think, "I'm fine now, I don't need it." But consistent upkeep is crucial.

How to Address Early Warning Signs

1. **Resume Your Basics**
   Go back to the simple methods that worked before. If breathing exercises or short breaks helped once, they can help again. Do not wait until the anxiety is overwhelming; use them early.
2. **Talk to Someone**
   A quick chat with a friend or a counselor can remind you of your tools. Sometimes, an outside perspective can spot a small fix that you missed.
3. **Adjust, Don't Give Up**
   If your old routine no longer fits your current life, tweak it. For instance, if journaling at night is not possible, try a quick morning note. Keep the essence, change the format.
4. **Use a Recap List**
   If you wrote down coping skills in earlier chapters (like calm breathing, self-talk, or scheduling breaks), keep that list where you can see it. Look at it when you sense anxiety rising.

Keeping Routines Fresh

After doing the same thing for a long time, boredom can set in. You might stop feeling the benefits. To keep routines effective:

1. **Rotate Exercises**
   Instead of the same breathing exercise daily, rotate among a few techniques. Try a muscle relaxation drill on Mondays, a slow breathing count on Tuesdays, etc. Variety keeps the mind engaged.
2. **Set Small Challenges**
   For example, if you have become comfortable with your current level of social activity, you might set a new goal to chat with two new people this week or volunteer for a local event. This step-by-step push keeps your growth active.
3. **Reward Yourself**
   Even small achievements—like doing a relaxation exercise three days in a row—can be followed by a treat, like reading a short chapter of a fun book or taking a relaxing bath. This keeps motivation alive.
4. **Involve a Friend**
   If you have a friend who also wants to manage stress, you can share your

weekly routines. Text each other updates or remind each other to do them. This social element can reenergize the process.

Long-Term Problem-Solving

1. **Identify Root Causes**
   Sometimes, short-term methods handle symptoms, but deeper issues remain. If your job is extremely stressful or a relationship is toxic, you might need to solve these core problems. That could mean finding new work, seeking couples counseling, or making bigger life changes.
2. **Refine Skills**
   Over time, you can move from basic techniques to more advanced ones. For instance, if you used simple thought replacement, you might look into deeper cognitive therapy methods to break long-standing negative patterns.
3. **Stay Flexible**
   What worked a year ago might not fit now. Maybe your schedule or environment changed. Regularly review your routines to make sure they match your current life.
4. **Seek Knowledge**
   Keep learning about mental health. New research or advice might offer fresh insights. Books, reputable websites, or short courses can expand your toolbox.

Coping with Major Life Events

1. **Plan for Big Changes**
   If you know a major event is coming—like moving, changing jobs, or having a child—expect some anxiety. Reinforce your coping methods in advance. Let trusted people know you might need extra support.
2. **Use a Step-by-Step Approach**
   Tackle big tasks in smaller parts. If moving homes, you might pack one room at a time. If starting a new job, you might practice new skills or read about the company slowly rather than all at once.
3. **Accept Temporary Instability**
   During big changes, your routine might be thrown off. You may feel

disorganized. This is normal. Once things settle, rebuild your stable habits.

4. **Request Help**
   For instance, if you are dealing with a health issue, ask a friend to drive you to appointments. If you are relocating, see if a relative can keep important items safe while you settle in. Leaning on others can reduce anxiety in transition periods.

Long-Term Medications or Therapy

Some people find they do well after a short time in therapy or on medication, while others need longer support. If you are on medication:

- **Schedule Checkups**
  Regularly meet with the prescribing professional to see if your dosage is still correct, or if you can safely reduce it.
- **Watch for Side Effects**
  Over time, side effects might change. Report any new issues right away.
- **Stay Honest with Therapists**
  If you feel therapy sessions have stopped being helpful, bring it up. You can adjust the focus or try a new approach.

If you do well without medication, that is also fine, as long as you keep track of anxiety signs. The key is to remain aware. It is possible to return to therapy or medication if new life stressors arise.

Balancing Self-Care and Responsibility

1. **Time Management**
   If you become busy, self-care can slip off the schedule. Making a simple plan—like setting aside 20 minutes daily to unwind—can keep it alive.
2. **Energy Guardrails**
   Know your energy limits. If you commit to too many social events or tasks, stress can build. Polite refusal when overloaded can save you from a meltdown later.
3. **Celebrate Others' Progress Too**
   Encouraging friends who also manage anxiety can remind you that

everyone grows at their own pace. Sharing a positive word can help both sides, as you reaffirm the value of the coping methods.
4. **Personal Growth Projects**
Working on something meaningful outside of anxiety management—like learning a new skill, improving finances, or building deeper relationships—keeps your mind from focusing only on worry. It gives a sense of purpose that can anchor you when stress arises.

Handling Surprises or Setbacks

1. **Allow Emotions**
If something triggers anxiety suddenly—like an unexpected bill—let yourself feel upset for a short time. Then try to shift into problem-solving mode: "What can I do about this right now?"
2. **Use Quick Calming Methods**
Deep breathing, a 5-minute walk, or a short phone call to a supportive friend can ground you. Responding early can prevent the worry from escalating.
3. **Reflect**
After the surprise passes, reflect on how you handled it. Did any new coping skill work well? Did you notice a gap in your plan? This reflection sharpens your approach for next time.
4. **Reassure Yourself of Past Wins**
Remind yourself of other times you overcame a surprise. This keeps you from feeling helpless and shows you that you are capable of managing unexpected events.

Maintaining Motivation

Over months and years, you might question if the effort is worth it. Some ways to stay motivated:

1. **Track Small Gains**
Keep a simple log or note each time you handle stress well. Even small successes—like calmly making a phone call or finishing a task without panic—count. Reviewing these can inspire you.

2. **Remember Your Original Pain**
   Think back to how bad anxiety felt before you started these methods. Reflect on how far you have come. This can remind you why you do not want to return to old patterns.
3. **Reward Patterns**
   If you complete your weekly routine for a month, treat yourself to something safe and enjoyable, like a new book or a relaxing activity. This sense of progress can push you forward.
4. **Visualize a Balanced Future**
   Imagine yourself calmly handling daily life or reaching personal goals without constant worry. This picture of a more peaceful life can act as a beacon that keeps you going.

Teaching Others

Sometimes, teaching or guiding others who struggle with anxiety can reinforce your own skills:

- **Share Simple Tools**
  Show a friend how to do a breathing exercise or how to track worry patterns. Explaining it can deepen your own understanding.
- **Offer Encouragement**
  If someone is behind you in this process, let them know it is normal to have setbacks. Telling them about your journey can remind you of your own growth.
- **Stay Humble**
  Teaching does not mean you never worry. It just means you have a few experiences to share. You can still learn from the person you are helping.
- **Prevent Overstretching**
  Be careful not to take on the role of their sole therapist. Encourage them to seek professional help if needed. Keep your own limits in mind so you do not become too stressed.

Periodic Self-Audits

Every few months, do a quick "self-audit" on your mental health:

1. **Rate Your Anxiety**
   On a scale of 1 to 10, how would you rate your anxiety in the past week?
2. **Check Routines**
   Are you still doing the helpful routines from earlier chapters, or have some slipped away?
3. **Review Life Areas**
   Look at work, relationships, health, and personal goals. Is anything there raising extra anxiety that you have not faced?
4. **Adjust**
   Based on what you find, make changes. If you have let bedtime slip, fix it. If you have avoided a certain chore, handle it. Small tweaks prevent bigger problems later.

Planning for the Long-Term Future

1. **Set Realistic Goals**
   If you want to continue your self-improvement, pick achievable aims. For example, "I want to speak up more in meetings," or "I want to deal with traffic stress better."
2. **Visualize Next Steps**
   Sketch out the steps needed for each goal. Maybe you read an article on public speaking or ask a coworker how they prepare notes. Then practice.
3. **Allow Space for Uncertainty**
   As discussed in the previous chapter, the future is not fully predictable. Keep an open mind, and do not rely on everything going perfectly.
4. **Integrate Maintenance into Life**
   Over time, see your anxiety-reducing habits as normal parts of your routine, not special tasks. For instance, morning stretches or evening journaling can be as natural as brushing your teeth.

Reinventing Your Identity

If you used to identify as "the anxious person," it might feel strange to see yourself as calmer. Let yourself adjust to this new identity. You can be someone who experiences worry but also has strong coping skills:

- **Avoid Over-Labeling**
  If you no longer have daily panic attacks, you might hesitate to use old negative labels. You are still you, just with better tools.
- **Accept Occasional Anxiety**
  It is normal to feel anxiety sometimes. The difference is now you do not let it run your life. That is real progress.
- **Focus on Other Traits**
  Anxiety is just one part of you. You might also be creative, funny, caring, good with details, or many other things. Balancing these traits in your identity can reduce the mental weight of anxiety.

Handling the "What-If" of Recurrence

You might worry, "What if my anxiety returns in full force?" Even if it does:

1. **Remember Your Skills**
   You have a toolbox now—breathing, scheduling, self-talk, support networks, and more. You can pull them out again.
2. **Seek Professional Guidance (If Needed)**
   If you see a big spike, do not hesitate to revisit a counselor or your doctor. Early intervention can keep it from escalating.
3. **Use a Progress Mindset**
   A relapse does not erase your previous work. You learned from it before, and you can apply that knowledge again to bounce back.
4. **Stay Hopeful**
   You have coped with anxiety in the past and made it this far. That is proof you can do so again. People rarely lose all progress permanently.

Looking Back, Looking Forward

Throughout these 20 chapters, you have explored anxiety from many angles. You learned about signs, causes, negative thought patterns, self-talk, stress management, diet, sleep, healthy routines, panic, social fears, workplace or school concerns, mindset, long-term strategies, medication and therapy, breaking harmful habits, finding personal strength, facing uncertainty, and giving and receiving support. Now you know that anxiety does not define who you are.

It is a condition that can be managed with consistent effort and a balanced approach.

Maintenance is the final piece. It ensures that all these strategies do not fade away. By keeping an eye on your signs, sticking with helpful routines, and being flexible as life changes, you can keep anxiety at a manageable level. It might still appear from time to time, but it will not rule your days like before. Instead, you will have calm, clarity, and the capacity to face challenges with more poise.

Final Thoughts

- **Stay Gentle with Yourself**
  Anxiety thrives on self-criticism. Practice kindness inwardly. Even if you miss a routine or slip into old habits, treat it as a temporary pause. Start again.
- **Celebrate Small Moments**
  You do not need fireworks to mark each success. Even a quick acknowledgment—"I faced that phone call and stayed calm"—nourishes your sense of progress.
- **Keep Growing**
  Anxiety management is not the end. It can be the start of a broader personal development path. You might find that, once free of the heaviest worry, you can explore passions or form better connections.
- **Share Your Story**
  Talking about your wins and lessons can lighten someone else's load. It also reminds you of what you overcame and how strong you have become.

Bringing It All to a Close

You have reached the end of this book, but the process of living with less anxiety continues. Each day, you have a choice: to use the steps you learned, to reach out for help, to support others, and to refine your mindset. Over time, these choices shape a calmer life, one in which anxiety may still exist but does not dominate. You have read about numerous methods, from eating better to setting healthy routines, from seeking therapy if needed to breaking old habits that fed your worry.

It is up to you to make these methods part of your routine. Some might fit more naturally, some less so. Experiment, adapt, and keep an open mind. If you run into blocks, look back on these chapters or seek new knowledge. Anxiety might be stubborn, but so is the human spirit. You have more power than you might think. This book aimed to show how many angles there are to address anxiety—body, mind, environment, habits, and relationships. Combining them can lead to real relief.

In closing, remember: nobody is perfect at this. Anxiety can still appear in stressful times. Yet each tool you have gathered can reduce its strength. Each time you notice anxious thoughts and choose a new response, you build confidence. Each time you open up to a friend or find a moment of calm, you reinforce the truth that you can handle life's demands. By maintaining progress—checking in regularly, staying flexible, and using your support system—you can create a steady path forward.

Life always has twists and turns, but with your improved self-awareness and coping skills, you are better equipped to meet those twists on your own terms. May the knowledge you have gained become a lasting resource, and may your days include more calm moments and fewer anxious storms. You have taken an important step in reading this book. Now, keep going with the practices that help you stay stable and content. You deserve a life where worry does not overshadow everything, and each chapter of your real-life story can reflect that growing sense of peace.

www.ingramcontent.com/pod-product-compliance
Lightning Source LLC
LaVergne TN
LVHW012105070526
838202LV00056B/5629